3 STEPS TO INCREDIBLE HEALTH!

VOLUME I

JOEL FUHRMAN, M.D.

PUBLISHED BY

ɋɧ

Gift of Health Press

OTHER BOOKS BY JOEL FUHRMAN, M.D.

Eat To Live

Eat For Health

Disease-Proof Your Child

Cholesterol Protection For Life

Fasting and Eating For Health

Published by Gift of Health Press, Flemington, New Jersey.

Contact:
Joel Fuhrman, M.D.
4 Walter Foran Boulevard, Suite 409
Flemington, NJ 08822

Publisher's Note:
Keep in mind that results vary from person to person. Some people have a medical
history and/or condition that may warrant individual recommendations and
in some cases drugs and even surgery. Do not start, stop, or change medication
without professional medical advice, and do not change your diet if you are ill or
on medication except under the supervision of a competent physician. Neither
this, nor any other book, is intended to take the place of personalized medical care
or treatment.

The names used in success stories have been changed.

Printed in the United States of America

Design: Robyn Rolfes, Creative Syndicate, Inc.
Cover Design: Savita Naidu
Cover Photograph: Sandra Nissen

Library of Congress Control Number: 2011925250

ISBN: 978-0-9799667-7-4

First Edition

DEDICATION

This book is dedicated to every American who is suffering with chronic disease, especially those who have been told that their problems are genetic and that drugs or invasive interventions are the only answers.

Even though the powerful therapeutic benefits of superior nutrition have been well documented in the scientific literature, this information has not been made available to the general public. Depriving people of the right to know that recoveries are possible through superior nutrition leads to needless suffering and—all too often—premature death.

People have a right to know that they have a choice. They have a right to know that they do not have to suffer and die prematurely from medical conditions that are easily prevented and reversed. If you think you deserve better health, if you want to reduce medical expenditures and avoid surgeries and medications, or if you just want to live longer—with good health and mental facilities intact, this book is dedicated to you with the hope that the menus, recipes, and other information presented will be of help to you as you transform your life.

CONTENTS

Preface

My reasons for writing this book are twofold. First and foremost, people are suffering and dying tragically and unnecessarily from diseases that they could easily prevent and easily recover from. I have been part of the medical community as a family physician for almost twenty years, and I want to tell you what almost every doctor knows: Drugs and doctors cannot grant you excellent health and protection from disease and suffering. The most effective health care is proper self-care.

In these pages, I will describe the steps necessary to learn, practice, and master the best possible self-care program—superior nutrition. Superior nutrition is built upon my high-nutrient diet. This approach is so successful that most people can prevent and even reverse most medical problems within three to six months. This is a bold claim, but the facts, supported by scientific research, show that most of the health problems and tragedies we face in the modern world are the result of nutritional folly. Your body has to build and rebuild itself from the foods you eat. When you eat the standard American diet (SAD), you get the standard American diseases. By age fifty, the majority of Americans are taking prescription drugs for one or more diseases.

I first described my high-nutrient approach to eating in my 2003 best-selling book, *Eat To Live* (revised in 2011), and I have received an avalanche of letters and e-mails of gratitude from people who have seen miraculous changes in their health as a result of dietary changes. Those testimonies—some of which you will read here—led to the second reason for writing this book. I needed to share the new lessons I was learning about the obstacles people encounter when making dietary changes. I want to give as many people as possible the chance to make the changes necessary to achieve incredible health.

I want to give *you* that chance.

Thirty-eight percent of Americans die of heart attacks and strokes. You don't have to be one of them. Twenty-eight million Americans suffer from the crippling pain of osteoarthritis. You don't have to be one of them. Thirty-five million Americans suffer from chronic headaches. You don't have to be one of them. You simply do not have to be sick.

It is considered "normal" to lose youthful vigor in your thirties, to gain thirty or forty extra pounds and live with chronic illness in your late forties and fifties, and become so debilitated that you live your last decades completely dependent on others. But this is not normal. This is the inevitable result of a lifelong pattern of unhealthful living based on misguided information. What is truly normal, outrageous as it may sound, is to look forward to enjoying a healthy, active life into your nineties. The reason it sounds outrageous is that most people spend their lifetimes consuming very unhealthful diets, and they don't make the connection between what they eat and the inevitable ill health that follows in their later years.

I have cared for more than 15,000 patients. Most of them came to my office unhappy, sick, and overweight, having tried every dietary craze without success. After following my educational program for superior health and weight loss, they shed the weight they always dreamed of losing... and they kept it off. For the first time in their lives, they had a diet plan that didn't require them to be hungry all the time. Most importantly, they were able to eventually discontinue their medications because they simply didn't need them anymore.

When you learn and follow this program of eating, it is possible to:

- never have a heart attack or stroke

- avoid dementia in later life

- dramatically reduce your chance of getting cancer

- prevent and heal digestive problems such as reflux, dyspepsia, constipation, and hemorrhoids

- prevent and often resolve erectile impotence, high blood pressure, and other circulatory impairments

- prevent and reverse diabetes (Type II) and high cholesterol, at first lessening the need for drugs and eventually resolving these conditions

- age more slowly, live longer, and maintain youthful vigor, intelligence, and productivity into your later years

Some people may be skeptical about these claims, but, rest assured, they are supported by medical science and thousands of clinical patient case histories. The reversal of dietary-caused diseases occurs in a relatively short time and is easily observed by anyone following my program. I believe that everyone has the right to know that they have a choice when it comes to protecting their precious health.

ACKNOWLEDGEMENTS

I had assistance from many people in developing this book. My wife, Lisa, reads everything I write and helps me immensely. My editors, Jim Lennon and Susan Taylor Lennon, have done another fantastic job. Robyn Rolfes designed the book, and Savita Naidu designed the diagrams and cover. Linda Popescu, R.D., worked with me on *Dr. Fuhrman's Nutrient Density Scores*, and Deana Ferrari, Ph.D., assisted with research. I want to thank members at DrFuhrman.com who shared their success stories. I appreciate their generosity and desire to help others. The contributions of my executive team, Janice McDonnell-Marra and Dominic Ambrosio, were invaluable. Finally, I want to thank my children—Talia, Jenna, Cara, and Sean—who serve as loyal taste-testers for my *unique* recipe ideas and who support me in so many ways.

Congratulations on taking your first steps toward incredible health! You are embarking on one of the most important journeys you will ever undertake. Twenty years of clinical practice in nutritional medicine and a lifetime of dedicated interest and study in human nutrition has convinced me that superior nutrition—centered around a high-nutrient, plant-based diet—is absolutely essential to high-quality health. In addition to my own research and observations, I have conducted an in-depth review of more than 20,000 scientific studies on human nutrition and translated that science into an easy-to-understand approach to eating that ensures both high-nutrient consumption and great tasting meals. You will be hearing the term "high-nutrient" quite a bit in this book. That's because high-nutrient foods and meals will be the recipe for your nutritional turnaround.

The results achieved by people following my dietary and lifestyle program are truly astonishing. In addition to preventing many common diseases, my approach can be a powerful intervention in the process of *reversing* them. I have seen its beneficial effects on thousands of patients with a wide range of diseases and health concerns, ranging from migraines and allergies to heart disease and diabetes. These health improvements are a tribute both to each patient's efforts and to the ever-increasing power of modern nutritional science to help patients completely recovery from most chronic degenerative illnesses.

Success stories

You will be reading testimonials from people who have transformed their lives following my recommendations. They have different ages, different backgrounds, and different reasons for making healthful changes in their lives. But now they all have one thing in common— excellent health. As you read their stories, think about the benefits that will become possible for you when you start to eat right and make a commitment to your health. Superior nutrition unleashes seemingly miraculous human health capabilities—including the potential to reverse chronic diseases—that are rarely understood or appreciated by health authorities or the medical profession.

I coined the term *high-nutrient diet* to emphasize this most important aspect of my dietary recommendations, the key component that sets it apart from other diets. My approach is unique because it is designed to optimize micronutrient density, micronutrient diversity, and micronutrient completeness. Attention is paid not just to vitamins and minerals, but to the thousands of other phytonutrients important for maximizing immune function, preventing cancer and other diseases, and increasing healthy longevity. Thousands of people around the world are eating my high-nutrient, plant-based diet and are enjoying healthier and more pleasurable lives.

Simply put, as you read and progress along the steps toward incredible health, you will develop a clear understanding of how striving for more micronutrients per calorie in your diet and consuming a broad array of micronutrients can bring powerful disease-protecting and therapeutic effects into your life. It is not sufficient to merely avoid fats, consume foods with a low glycemic index, lower the intake of animal products, or eat a diet with lots of raw foods. A truly healthful diet must be micronutrient-rich, and the micronutrient richness must be adjusted to meet your individual needs. The foods with the highest micronutrient-per-calorie ratios are vegetables, and for optimal health and to combat disease, it is necessary to consume sufficient quantities of them.

Your body has a tremendous capacity for self-healing when you provide it with an optimal nutritional environment. You soon will know the most effective way to create that environment. If you have high blood pressure, high cholesterol, diabetes, heart disease, indigestion, headaches, asthma, fatigue, body aches, or pain, or simply want to prevent them, this book is for you. My high-nutrient diet can enable you to avoid angioplasty, bypass surgery, and other invasive procedures, and virtually ensure that you will never suffer a heart attack or stroke or develop dementia. You can reduce and eventually eliminate your need for prescription drugs. You can optimize your health and potentially save your life.

Lose weight naturally

For most people, weight loss is a welcome side effect of improved diet and lifestyle habits. Rest assured, on my high-nutrient diet you will lose all the weight you want, even if diets have failed you in the past. A recent medical study confirmed that the nutritional program presented in this book is the most effective weight-loss plan ever documented in medical literature, especially if you have a lot of weight to lose.[1] After two years, participants lost more weight than the subjects of any other study in medical history, and they kept it off. Additional medical studies also have demonstrated that diets rich in high-nutrient plant foods have a suppressive effect on appetite and are most effective for long-term weight control.[2] So it should come as no surprise that the healthiest way to eat is also the most successful way to obtain and maintain a favorable weight.

My unique discovery in the field of nutritional science is related directly to my high-nutrient diet. My paper, "Changing perceptions of hunger on a high-nutrient-density diet," which was published in *Nutrition Journal,* documents that as people increase the micronutrient quality of their diet, it lessens their hunger and curtails their desire to overeat.[3] This discovery helps to explain the dramatic weight-loss success of this program. (For those interested in reading the entire paper online, a web link is included with the reference.)

As effective as it is for weight loss (patients have lost up to twenty pounds in six weeks, and that was just the beginning), *3 Steps to Incredible Health* is not a "diet book" in the traditional sense. It describes a way of eating that you will adopt for the rest of your life, not just for three weeks so that you can look slimmer at your daughter's wedding. There is no calorie counting, no portion-size measuring, and no weighing involved. You will eat as much food as you want. Eating healthfully for the long term is more effective for weight control than "dieting" because it modifies and diminishes the sensations of so-called hunger, enabling overweight individuals to be more comfortable eating fewer calories. Reaching your ideal weight will be a pleasant and automatic by-product that occurs naturally on the road to maximizing your health.

High-nutrient density

Most people do not consume enough micronutrients. Because their micronutrient needs aren't met, they can't control food cravings and overeating. Typically, these people satisfy their food cravings by eating high-calorie, low-nutrient foods. Over time, this ongoing micronutrient deficiency makes them more susceptible to the diseases and serious medical conditions that are plaguing Americans—allergies, asthma, acne, headaches, high blood pressure, diabetes, reflux esophagitis, lupus, kidney insufficiency, angina, cardiomyopathy, multiple sclerosis, and many more.

Micronutrients consist of vitamins, minerals, and phytochemicals—valuable, calorie-free elements contained in certain foods. My high-nutrient diet program dramatically reduces your consumption of low-nutrient foods and just as dramatically increases your intake of high-nutrient foods. The program will never ask you to count calories, but for good health and a long, disease-free life, you need to plan your eating around foods that have a high nutrient-to-calorie ratio. In other words, foods that are higher in micronutrients and lower in calories. To make it easy for you, later in the book I will show you how to choose foods that have the highest nutrient density (and provide a list). In addition, I have written a companion book, *3 Steps to Incredible Health, Volume 2,* that includes over 150 delicious, high-nutrient recipes and three levels of menus to make it easy for you to follow the recommendations in this book.

Adequate consumption of vitamins, minerals, and phytochemicals is essential for a healthy immune system, and these micronutrients are necessary to empower the detoxification and cellular repair mechanisms that protect you from cancer and other diseases. Perhaps not surprisingly, you will find that most of the foods that have a high-nutrient density are fruits and vegetables. These foods will play major roles in your journey to great health. Over the last twenty years, nutritional science has demonstrated that colorful plant foods contain a huge assortment of protective compounds, most of which are still being discovered and studied by scientists. We are learning that these compounds work in fascinating ways to detoxify carcinogens, repair DNA damage, reduce free radical formation, and facilitate the removal of toxins from the body. Only by eating an assortment of nutrient-rich, natural plant foods can you obtain the diversity of elements needed to protect yourself from common diseases.

Three steps to incredible health

This book is divided into three sections to correspond with the three steps to incredible health. Section 1 teaches you the power of micro-nutrients. Learning to make high-nutrient foods the foundation of your diet is the first step toward superior health. Section 2 teaches you how to overcome your food addictions and unnatural desire to overeat. This second step starts you on the road toward renewed self-esteem and health independence. Section 3 teaches you how to use super foods to develop super health. This third step begins your total health transformation. Here, you embark on a new, evermore healthful and pleasurable way of eating, and you virtually disease-proof yourself at the same time.

Making substantive dietary changes can seem like an insurmount-able challenge, and the addiction to certain foods can be just as deadly as many other addictions. Don't worry. I will show you how to get rid of the food addictions that are sabotaging your health. The secret to success rests on your willingness to discard the out-of-date, limiting beliefs held by most Americans and embrace the possibility that you will discover a level of enjoyment in eating that you have never imag-ined. It all begins with a new state of mind.

You will be presented with logical, scientific information that explains the connection between diet and health. These facts may require you to change the way you think about food. I suggest that you read the material completely before making any big dietary decisions. That way, you will be in an educated position as you decide what and when to change. If you are relatively healthy, you can go at your own pace. If you have health concerns, I suggest that you make substantial dietary changes more quickly.

The reason this program works so well is because its success is built on knowledge and a step-by-step approach. It takes time and effort to learn this body of knowledge, since modern scientific nutrition contra-dicts the health misinformation to which we are accustomed. But once you have learned and practiced this information, you will be ready to begin the ultimate journey to the fullest enjoyment of your health. Experience has shown that the program works best for those who understand it best.

As you adopt this new way of eating, you will find that you truly enjoy and prefer it. This book will guide you through your transition as you step up to long lasting, excellent health. Along the way, you will create new, health-enhancing behaviors that will eventually become effortless. It is so highly effective that before long, you won't have to give a second thought to your weight, and your health destiny will be firmly in your own hands.

Getting started

The first few chapters cover the fundamentals of superior nutrition. You will learn to overcome the obstacles that are preventing you from adopting a healthful eating program for life. As you progress through the book, you will prepare for your new way of eating by doing my "Exercises with Food." As you move through the book, you will learn about my three levels of high-nutrient eating. Starting with Level 1, each level incorporates progressively higher nutritional principles that lead to a new disease-proof you. Level 3 is the most effective for reversing disease and maximizing health and longevity. If you are struggling with an autoimmune disease, cancer, or other serious illness, you will want to target Level 3 as your optimal diet. Otherwise, I find that Level 2 provides an excellent level of nutrient density for most of my patients. Level 1 can be a good place to start and a place to go when circumstances prevent you from getting a higher-level meal. All levels can help most people move closer to their health goals, and, if you are overweight, you will get dramatic benefits from all levels.

There are weekly menu plans for each level in *3 Steps to Incredible Health, Volume 2,* so you can pick a level and stay with it, or start at Level 1 and gradually progress to Levels 2 and 3. The menu plans allow you the option of moving back and forth between levels, making small but significant additions or subtractions to your diet. It may be that the change from the way you eat now to Level 1 will be a significant one. If so, you can make this first big change and stop there for a while. It's all up to you.

As you learn more and experiment with high-nutrient eating, your taste buds will gradually realign themselves and actually become stronger and more discriminating. As you become healthier, you will lose your psychological dependence on unhealthful foods. One of the ways in which the level-by-level approach can be of benefit is that the gradual implementation of increasingly higher micronutrient levels allows your taste buds to acclimate to the new diet. As you increase your knowledge and your preference for healthful foods grows, you can move forward—all at your own pace.

I feel strongly that this is the most healthful diet for disease-protection and longevity, and, if you are significantly overweight, it is also the safest and most effective way to lose a dramatic amount of weight. It works even for those who have failed at losing weight in the past. Studies have shown that only 3 percent of people who attempt to lose weight actually succeed. The problem is not the people. The problem is that most weight-loss approaches focus on reducing calories. That winds up reducing nutrients simultaneously, which is predictive of eventual failure. The approach in 3 Steps to Incredible Health is radically different from other plans because you get to eat a lot of food. Forget calorie counting and traditional diets. You will lose weight. As you increase your intake of nutrient-dense foods and eliminate unhealthful foods, you will begin to reset your internal taste preferences and hunger drive. Once this happens, you will be amazed at how easy it becomes to eat well, enjoy it, and maintain your ideal weight and health forever.

One word of caution

This program is so effective at dropping your weight, blood pressure, and blood sugar that medication adjustments will be necessary so that you are not overmedicated. If your blood sugar or blood pressure improves dramatically and medications are not reduced or eliminated, it could be harmful to your health. Please consult with your physician.

Finding Your Motivation

You are what you eat. To be your best, you must eat the best. Perhaps you already know this, but it is not always easy to do. I will teach you new nutritional principles to enable you to think and eat healthfully, but before you get started, you must find your motivation.

On a scale of 1 to 10, rate the most compelling reasons you have for eating healthfully:

_____ I want to recover from a chronic illness, such as high blood pressure, diabetes, headaches, or high cholesterol.

_____ I want to protect myself from developing a dangerous disease.

_____ I want to prevent the deterioration in health, physical, and mental abilities that are typically considered a normal part of aging.

_____ I want to lose weight and look and feel better.

_____ I want to increase my energy and reduce fatigue.

_____ I want to improve the health of my family.

_____ I want to improve my physical fitness.

_____ I want protection from frequent bouts of infectious disease.

_____ I want to have better digestion.

_____ I want to have better sexual enjoyment and performance.

_____ I want to look and feel younger.

_____ I want to have a better emotional outlook on life.

_____ I want to live longer.

_____ I want to live without medical interference and hospitalizations.

_____ I want to avoid surgery or prescription medication.

_____ I want to reduce my dependency on medication.

_____ I want to save money on health care and prescription drugs.

Each time you feel some difficulty in maintaining your new high-nutrient diet, each time you want to revert back to your old ways of eating, each time you slip up on the program, each time you believe the level of health you want is unattainable, come back and look at this page. Habits are hard to break, and you probably have many eating habits you need to break. Remind yourself of how important the things on this list are and why they are more than adequate motivation for continuing to learn, practice, and live with the goal of superior nutrition for optimal health.

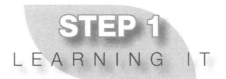

STEP 1
LEARNING IT

THE POWER OF MICRONUTRIENTS

Before we take *Step 1* and start learning about the Power of Micronutrients, I'd like to give you a little peek at the kind of success you can expect to achieve. I often find that people's success stories—people just like you—can be more motivating than scientific data alone. During the twenty years that I have been recommending the fundamentals of the high-nutrient diet to patients in my medical practice and to readers of my books, I have seen remarkable results in those who have followed my recommendations. The transformative power of adopting a dietary program centered around high-nutrient foods is astonishing. You could call it miraculous… except that it happens all the time.

Below is a sampling of the thousands of e-mails and letters that I have received from my patients and readers of my books (especially *Eat to Live*, where I first introduced my high-nutrient approach). These are individuals who have followed my nutritional advice and discovered that they could dramatically improve their weight, health, and enjoyment of life. Their illnesses and weight problems vary greatly, but they all have discovered that the power of superior nutrition is vastly superior to the power of prescription medicine. Browse through their stories, and let their personal experiences inform and motivate you in your quest for incredible health.

CLARISSA — HIGH BLOOD PRESSURE AND WEIGHT LOSS

I hadn't always struggled with my weight. In my thirties, I was thin, single, worked out every day, and ran three or four miles several times each week. But after getting married and having kids, the weight started creeping on. Although I joined two weight-loss organizations, I struggled with sugar. Once, I lost a lot of weight on the Atkins Diet, only to gain it right back—and then some. For ten years, I pretty much quit trying to get healthy and just stayed my same overweight self. I felt like hiding. I didn't want to participate in physical activities because it was too much effort, and I was always tired.

But that was before I read Dr. Fuhrman's *Eat to Live* book. I've followed his program for over a year now, and I feel like I have my life back! I no longer have sugar cravings, and I have lots of energy and confidence. I feel like the "real" me is here again because I'm not embarrassed by how I look anymore, and I'm not afraid to try new activities. This past summer, I climbed Sleeping Bear Dunes in northern Michigan with my family and went horseback riding with my daughter.

I've lost 50 pounds. I've gone from size 16 down to size 6. My cholesterol dropped 60 points, and I no longer have acid reflux disease, for which I had taken medication for twenty years. I'm still taking blood pressure medication, but I'm hopeful that soon I'll be off of that entirely. I'll turn fifty-seven this month, and I feel like I'm no longer getting older—I'm getting better!

MATHEW — ASTHMA, HIGH CHOLESTEROL, AND HIGH BLOOD PRESSURE

I was forty-nine, overweight (249 pounds), and sick—but in denial. Being over six foot three, the extra weight wasn't so noticeable. But because I was athletic when I was young, it was hard for me to accept that I was tired all the time, I was on four prescription medications for asthma, and I always had a runny nose. I always overate, and my diet was deadly. I would wake up during the night needing my inhaler just so I could breathe. I was worried that if I didn't do something quickly, my two daughters would lose their father to a heart attack or some other disease.

I started doing a lot of reading, and I discovered Dr. Fuhrman's *Eat to Live* book. After following his program, I started feeling great, I got off my medications, and the weight started to drop. Gone were the days of lethargy. In fact, two years after starting the program, I began training and ran my first marathon, the Marine Corps Marathon. It was pretty emotional for me when the Marine officer (I'm a former Marine) placed that medal around my neck as I reflected on how much I was enjoying my new life of health! The high-nutrient program didn't just heal me physically; it increased my self-esteem and gave me a different outlook on my future.

Five years into the program, I am the same weight that I was in high school (185 pounds). My cholesterol has dropped from 162 to 120, and my blood pressure has dropped from 144/95 to 118/75. Dr. Fuhrman's program has changed my entire outlook on life. After years of worrying about a heart attack, these thoughts are now gone. Every day seems brighter when you have your health!

VIRGINIA — PERIMENOPAUSE AND FERTILITY

I was six months shy of my fortieth birthday and 80 pounds overweight. My menstrual cycles were completely out of whack. Some months, they lasted for weeks, and some months they never came. I haphazardly attributed this to my age and family history of early menopause and grudgingly accepted that I most likely was not going to have children. Two physicians told me that my chances of conceiving naturally were extremely slim. It wasn't a complete surprise. A few years earlier, an endocrinologist had told me that I was perimenopausal and recommended that I begin hormone therapy, and a fertility specialist had told me that I had a limited number of eggs and highly recommended in vitro fertilization immediately. Thankfully, I didn't follow through with these suggestions.

A friend of mine suggested that I read Dr. Fuhrman's book, *Eat to Live*. I dove right into it that same day. I started to feel better right away. Lots of beneficial changes started taking place, but I was so focused on losing weight that I hardly noticed when I had three consecutive regular monthly cycles. It dawned on me that I was healing my body from the inside out, and this had everything to do with what I was putting into my mouth. Long gone were the days of chicken tenders, steak, fries, and pizza.

On my fortieth birthday, I told my husband that I thought I was healthy enough now to have children. And I was right! I got pregnant almost immediately, and on May 24, 2010, my beautiful and healthy daughter, Clara, was born.

Not long afterwards, I finally met Dr. Fuhrman, and I couldn't wait to share my story with him. I told him how he saved my life, how he made me healthy, and, best of all, how he helped me get pregnant!

My pregnancy was a dream—no morning sickness, gestational diabetes, preclampsia, or any other problems. Every single woman in my family suffered from these things, but I didn't!

Morris — Multiple Sclerosis

I was diagnosed with multiple sclerosis (MS) about four years ago. The first symptom occurred two years before that. The neurologist tried to reassure me by saying that MS was not a death sentence, and that only about one in twenty patients eventually require wheelchairs. I told him that I would not be one of them. I began taking Copaxone, but after the sixth day, I decided it was not the right thing for me. I started looking for alternative treatments.

I heard about Dr. Fuhrman and made an appointment. When he told me on that first visit that MS was not a problem and that we could handle it, my wife broke down in tears. Dr. Fuhrman explained everything, gave me a diet to follow, and that was that. I have only had one follow-up visit with him because I have steadily improved (no more numbness when I bend my neck, no more touching cold things on my legs and feeling like they are hot). I have absolutely no symptoms.

Since then, I have sent many people to Dr. Fuhrman, some with MS and some with lupus. They all are doing better. I regularly buy his books by the case and give them as gifts.

THE SCIENTIFIC SECRET TO SUCCESS

As we take *Step 1* together and start learning about the Power of Micronutrients, I hope that you are encouraged and inspired after reading the first group of success stories. It is important that you know that my high-nutrient dietary program is the only proven way to shed pounds, reverse existing diseases, and protect against future health problems. In the following pages, you will learn about the scientific foundation that supports this predictable success, and you will have an opportunity to make it part of your own life.

As I mentioned, the success stories are only a tiny sampling from the many thousands I have received from people whose lives have changed dramatically after adopting my program of high-nutrient eating. For example, so many of my patients have recovered from lupus and other autoimmune diseases that one of them interviewed the others and wrote a book about it. Skeptics may say that case histories of documented cases of disease recoveries are not sufficient and that medical studies are needed to corroborate these results.

I agree that more scientific studies would be helpful, and my colleagues and I are involved with several new research trials. However, some very important research supporting these concepts has been done already, so my case studies are not the only evidence that diseases such as high blood pressure, heart and circulatory diseases, diabetes, head-aches, and digestive problems can be prevented and resolved via better nutrition. These studies are referenced throughout the book, but let's briefly review a small sampling of them now.

Cardiovascular disease

The dietary recommendations described in this book and the elements that make a diet cardio-protective have been tested in multiple studies. The evidence is overwhelming. Let's first look at the LDL cholesterol-lowering effects of various dietary plans, as documented in published medical journal articles.

METHOD	DECREASE IN LDL CHOLESTEROL
American Heart Association standard low-fat advice[4]	6%
High protein (Atkins-type)[5]	No significant change
Low-fat vegetarian[6]	16%
Mediterranean[7]	No significant change
Cholesterol-lowering medication (statins)[8]	26%
High-nutrient-density[9]	33%

The high-nutrient diet includes many different qualities that make it cardio-protective and cholesterol-reducing. It's not just a low-fat or vegetarian way of eating that makes a diet ideal. This high-nutrient diet results in dramatic benefits because it is very high in mixed fibers and vegetables and has sterols and other compounds from beans and nuts. This is the only dietary intervention shown to lower cholesterol as effectively as cholesterol-lowering medications. Though the low-fat vegetarian diet lowered LDL cholesterol 16 percent, triglycerides were actually 18.7 percent higher and the LDL/HDL ratio remained unchanged. The results of the study that patterned the recommendations of the high-nutrient diet differed in that the LDL cholesterol was more significantly lowered without unfavorable impact on HDL or triglycerides, reflecting sizable improvement in cardiac risk factors. I have thousands of patients in my medical practice who have witnessed dramatic reductions in their blood lipids, especially LDL cholesterol, without drugs.

Keep in mind that cholesterol lowering does not adequately explain the protective effect of the high-nutrient diet in cardiovascular disease since the diet has powerful anti-inflammatory and other beneficial biochemical effects. Even though drugs may lower cholesterol, they cannot be expected to offer the dramatic protection against cardiovascular events that superior nutrition can.

The aggressive use of cholesterol-lowering drugs does not prevent most heart attacks and strokes and does not decrease the risk of fatal strokes.[10] In clinical trials, a significant percentage of patients on the best possible statin therapy still experience events. Lowering cholesterol through superior nutrition, however, can be expected to offer dramatically more protection and disease reversal compared to drug therapy, without the risk or expense of prescription medication. Consider these medical journal articles:

1) The effect of a plant-based diet on plasma lipids in hypercholesterolemic adults: a randomized trial. *Annals of Internal Medicine* (2005)

This study showed that when two diets have the same amount of fat and saturated fat, it is the one with the higher amount of high-nutrient plant material that gives the best results for cholesterol-lowering and other measurable disease risks. Here is the conclusion:

> "Previous national dietary guidelines primarily emphasized avoiding saturated fat and cholesterol; as a result, the guidelines probably underestimated the potential LDL cholesterol-lowering effect of diet. In this study, emphasis on including nutrient-dense plant-based foods, consistent with recently revised national guidelines, increased the total and LDL cholesterol-lowering effect of a low-fat diet."[11]

2) The combination of high fruit and vegetable and low saturated fat intakes is more protective against mortality in aging men than is either alone: the Baltimore Longitudinal Study of Aging. *The Journal of Nutrition* (2005)

This study showed that reducing saturated fat intake is helpful in reducing heart disease deaths, but in terms of the potential to reduce death from all causes, it is not as effective as diets that are high in fresh vegetables and fruits. The study showed, however, that when there is a low saturated fat intake and a higher intake of vegetables, fruits, and beans, the benefits are dramatic. Over an eighteen-year follow-up of more than 501 initially healthy men, researchers found that when both parameters were met, men consuming more than five servings of fruits and vegetables per day and getting less than 12 percent of calories from saturated fat were 76 percent less likely to die of heart disease and 31 percent less likely to die from all-cause mortality (meaning all causes of death). The study stated:

> "These findings demonstrate that the combination of both behaviors is more protective than either alone, suggesting that their beneficial effects are mediated by different mechanisms."[12]

3) Plant-based foods and prevention of cardiovascular disease: an overview. *American Journal of Clinical Nutrition* (2003)

This study concluded:

> "Evidence from prospective cohort studies indicates that a high consumption of plant-based foods such as fruit and vegetables, nuts, and whole grains is associated with a significantly lower risk of coronary artery disease and stroke. The protective effects of these foods are probably mediated through multiple beneficial nutrients contained in these foods, including antioxidant vitamins, minerals, phytochemicals, fiber, and plant proteins. In dietary practice, healthful plant-based diets do not necessarily have to be low in fat. Instead, these diets should include unsaturated fats as the predominant form of dietary fat, such as nuts. Such diets, which also have many other health benefits, deserve more emphasis in dietary recommendations to prevent chronic diseases."[13]

These studies are representative of thousands that illustrate that superior nutrition could have profound effects on each of us and on the collective health of our nation. In my many years of medical practice caring for thousands of patients with advanced and even unstable heart disease, every one of the patients who adopted my nutritional advice for the long term improved their cardiac condition. Not one has experienced another heart attack. Many physicians using aggressive nutritional interventions for patients with heart disease, including Caldwell Esselstyn, M.D., and Dean Ornish, M.D., have documented similar results. For example, Dr. Esselstyn followed seventeen very ill patients with documented, advanced triple-vessel disease on angiography over a sixteen-year period. The patients recovered, their angina resolved, and they got well. He stated, "In this study, patients become virtually heart-attack proof, which is remarkable since these same patients had experienced 48 cardiac events among them in the eight years prior to joining the study."[14]

The evidence conclusively shows that the national dietary guidelines, and even the improved recommendations of the American Heart Association, do not go far enough to offer people the information necessary for maximizing results.

Modern cardiology is focused on drugs and high-tech interventions that do little to extend life span. However, for those desiring more than mediocrity and true protection against heart disease and premature death, there is a clear-cut answer. The most effective and safest way to lower your LDL cholesterol and protect your long-term health is to adopt the high-nutrient diet.

Diabetes

As the number of people with Type II (adult onset) diabetes continues to soar, it is openly recognized that the growing waistline of the modern world is the main cause of this epidemic. Most physicians, dietitians, and even the American Diabetes Association have virtually given up on weight reduction as the primary treatment for diabetics. Consider this statement from a medical advisory committee: "It is nearly impossible to take very obese people and get them to lose significant weight. So rather than specifying an amount of weight loss, we are targeting getting metabolic control." This is doublespeak for "Our recommended diets don't work, so we just give medications and watch patients gradually deteriorate as the diabetes advances."

Today, medications are the mainstay of treatment and, unfortunately, most of these medications cause weight gain, worsening the syndrome and making the individual more diabetic. Additionally, the narrow focus on blood-sugar reduction and reliance on medications gives patients a false sense of security because they mistakenly think their somewhat better controlled glucose levels are an indication of restored or improved health. They continue to gain weight since they are following the same dietary habits that originally caused the problem.

It is well accepted that the most successful approach would be for people to stick with weight reduction and high-nutrient eating. Patients with diabetes who successfully lose weight from undergoing gastric bypass surgery typically see their diabetes melt away.[15] Dietary programs that have been successful at affecting weight loss have been dramatically effective for diabetics, too, enabling patients to discontinue medications.[16]

Preventing and reversing diabetes is not all about weight loss. The nutritional features of the high-nutrient diet have profound effects on improving pancreatic function and lowering insulin resistance over and above what could be accomplished through weight loss alone. The increased fiber, micronutrients, and stool bulk, plus the cholesterol-lowering and anti-inflammatory effects of this diet, have dramatic effects on Type II diabetes. Scores of my patients have been able to restore their glucose levels to the normal range without any further need for medications. They have become nondiabetic. Even my thin, Type I insulin-dependent diabetic patients typically are able to reduce their insulin requirements by almost half and have better glucose control using this high-nutrient approach.

Diets high in fiber and vegetables consistently have been shown to be beneficial for diabetic patients and offer considerably better results when compared with the current recommendations of the American Diabetes Association Diet.[17] The dietary advice typically offered to diabetics is not science-based; it caters to food preferences and food addictions. In contrast, my program describes a dietary approach that maximizes benefits for weight reduction, cardio-protection, and diabetes reversal.

Autoimmune disease

Working with patients who have autoimmune diseases is one of the most rewarding aspects of my medical practice. Autoimmune and immune-mediated illnesses include diseases such as rheumatoid arthritis, lupus, psoriasis, multiple sclerosis, connective tissue disease, and the inflammatory bowel diseases called ulcerative colitis and Crohn's, but there are also more than 100 clinical syndromes considered autoimmune diseases. Obviously, not every patient with these diseases can make a complete, drug-free recovery; however, the amazing thing is that so many patients can, and do, recover. The recoveries are not limited to recognized autoimmune diseases. I see many patients with pain syndromes without laboratory documentation of autoimmune disease. The ability to achieve substantial improvement, and, in many cases, complete remission of these supposedly incurable illnesses, is exciting.

I have been writing about these success stories for many years, including submissions to medical journals.[18] For the past twenty years, multiple studies have been published documenting the effectiveness of high-vegetable diets on autoimmune illnesses.[19] These largely have been ignored by the medical profession, and most doctors still deny the effectiveness of nutrition on autoimmune and inflammatory conditions. Nonetheless, the book you have in your hands describes the critical features of the diet most effective in aiding people suffering with these conditions. Although it is not clear why the studies showing the effectiveness of diet are quickly forgotten or ignored after their publication, one factor may be that there is no financial incentive for anyone to promote the power of dietary intervention as a medical therapy. However, pharmaceutical companies make large profits when studies show some efficacy for their products.

TO BE HEALTHY, EAT HEALTHY

The high-nutrient dietary program is not like any you've heard about before. The entire thought process behind it differs from conventional diets. When I first developed my approach of healing, I started by asking, "What is the healthiest way to eat?" The program described in this book, which I have perfected over the years, is the answer. The fact that it is also the most effective way to lose weight is a great bonus. Other diets and nutrition plans seem to be based on the premise, "How can we make a popular diet, and what type of gimmick will sell books?" My primary goal in writing and teaching about nutrition has never been popularity or economic success. As a doctor, I have a duty to patients who rely on me for lifesaving advice. My goal has been to be scientifically accurate and to create an eating program that is most effective for both weight loss and disease reversal.

Superior nutrition was, and still is, the answer. One of the most radical adjustments you have to make in following the high-nutrient diet is forgetting what you consider a normal portion size. Typical portion sizes are far too small for this plan. Get ready to discover that eating much larger amounts of the right foods—high-nutrient foods—is the secret to long-term weight loss and great health.

Once you focus on increasing your consumption of healthful foods, you will find that you aren't as hungry for the unhealthful foods you previously preferred. It's up to you when to start reducing your consumption of these foods. The sooner, the better, obviously, because the sooner you make the change, the sooner you will see dramatic results. But any changes you make that follow this plan will improve your health, weight, and wellness.

The first step towards achieving great health and maintaining your ideal weight forever is eating healthfully. Eating healthfully is all about eating more healthful foods. It sounds simple, right? It's not a brilliant or original idea, but most people don't understand which foods are truly healthful. Lots of people think a diet designed around pasta, chicken, and olive oil is healthful. Why? Because they say so on TV. But are these actually healthful foods? The answer is no, or at least not in the quantities that the average American consumes them. These foods are not rich in nutrients.

What determines the healthfulness of a food is how many nutrients it delivers to your body. In other words, for optimal health, you must eat foods that are truly rich in nutrients, and in particular, foods that deliver the greatest amount of nutrients for each calorie. This can be a strange concept for many people because they are accustomed to judging foods based on how many calories, fat grams, or carbohydrates they have. Try to wipe those ingrained ideas from your mind. With my plan, your primary concern will be the nutrients in the foods you eat. However, to eat this way, you must first understand what nutrients are and which foods have the greatest amounts of them.

Knowing your nutrients

There are two kinds of nutrients: *macro*nutrients and *micro*nutrients. Macronutrients are protein, carbohydrate, and fat. They contain calories. Micronutrients are vitamins, minerals, and phytochemicals. They are calorie-free. For ideal health, we need to consume both kinds of nutrients, but the American diet contains too many macronutrients and not enough micronutrients.

MACRONUTRIENTS = PROTEIN, CARBOHYDRATE, AND FAT*

Contain calories

Should limit consumption

* Water is also a macronutrient, omitted for this discussion

MICRONUTRIENTS = VITAMINS, MINERALS, AND PHYTOCHEMICALS

Do not contain calories

Should increase consumption

Eating foods that are rich in micronutrients is essential to achieving optimal health. A micronutrient-heavy diet supplies your body with 14 different vitamins, 25 different minerals, and more than 1,000 phytochemicals, which are plant-based chemicals that have profound effects on human cell function and the immune system. Foods that are naturally rich in these nutrients are also rich in fiber and water and are naturally low in calories, meaning they have a low caloric density. These low-calorie, high-nutrient foods provide the ingredients that enable your body's self-healing and self-repairing mechanisms. They are nature's contribution to your health turnaround!

In addition to eating more of these micronutrient-rich foods, you need to eat fewer macronutrients. Every nutritional scientist in the world agrees that moderate caloric restriction slows the aging process, prevents the development of chronic diseases, and extends life span. This has been tested in every species of animal, including primates. There is no controversy; Americans are eating themselves to death with too many calories. To change this, we must do three things:

EAT LESS FAT.   EAT LESS PROTEIN.   EAT LESS CARBOHYDRATE.

Although these reductions will be part of our focus, the high-nutrient diet is not primarily about calorie restriction. Simply trying to reduce calories is called dieting, and dieting doesn't work. The reason the high-nutrient program is so successful is because over time, without even trying or noticing it, you will prefer to eat fewer calories. I know that may sound unlikely. Many people think, "Not me, my body doesn't work that way," or, "It will be a real struggle for me." However, if you follow the program, it will happen instinctually. I have seen it happen to thousands of people, with all kinds of backgrounds and eating histories. I promise it can happen for you, too.

The key ingredient of the high-nutrient approach is this: You achieve superior health by eating more nutrient-rich foods and fewer high-calorie, low-nutrient foods. It works because the more high-nutrient food you consume, the less low-nutrient food you desire. Since the desire for these unhealthful foods will naturally diminish, all you need to do is focus on learning how to enjoy eating more high-nutrient food.

Foods are nutrient-dense when they contain a high level of micronutrients per calorie. Vegetables win the award for the most nutrient-dense foods on the planet. Therefore, as you move forward in your quest for superior nutrition, you will eat more and more vegetables. Vegetables have the most powerful association with protection from heart disease and cancer because they contain the most nutrients per calorie. This program will show you why a year-round consumption of high-nutrient, plant-based foods is the secret to obtaining superior health and your ideal weight. The recipes in *3 Steps to Incredible Health, Volume 2* will show you new and delicious ways to include many more vegetables in your daily menus.

Is this a vegetarian diet?

Vegetables and other high-nutrient foods are cornerstones of a high-nutrient diet, but this is not a book about becoming a strict vegetarian. Rather, its focus is on eating lots of anticancer super foods and significantly restricting the consumption of low-nutrient foods, including both processed foods and animal products. The high-nutrient way to health, longevity, and weight control differentiates itself from flexitarian or vegetarian paths because those approaches focus on the amount, frequency, and/or lack of animal products. The high-nutrient diet is defined by the consumption of lots of high-nutrient, healthful foods such as green vegetables, beans, onions, mushrooms, fruits, and seeds. Reducing the amount of animal products consumed (including down to zero, if you prefer) is primarily a function of reducing the amount of low-nutrient foods and avoiding processed foods. Whether or not you become a vegetarian or vegan is up to you. It is worth noting that typical vegetarian and vegan diets suffer as much from the overconsumption of low-nutrient foods and under-consumption of high-nutrient foods as do conventional diets.

The high-nutrient diet also is characterized by the avoidance of sugar and other sweeteners, white flour, refined oils, and processed foods in general. A high-nutrient diet affords many benefits for the individual and society in general by encouraging more people to take better care of their health through dietary improvements. Most people have some idea that eating better and eating more nutrient-rich foods will benefit them, but they don't know what those foods are, and they don't recognize the benefits and obstacles to adopting a healthful diet. You may already be eating a high-nutrient to some degree. This program will make it easier for you to fully embrace this dietary approach and accomplish your goals.

Healthful food choices at your door

Historically, a year-round diet that included a lot of vegetables and fruits simply wasn't possible. People were limited to foods that were grown locally and seasonally, so grains that could be stored for long periods became staples of most people's diets. However, grains are on the lower end of the nutrient density scale.

Nowadays, it is always growing season somewhere. Improvements in transportation and refrigeration have made it possible to move, freeze, and store fresh foods. This has given us year-round access to the healthiest and most nutrient-dense foods on the planet and an unprecedented opportunity to achieve and maintain superior health.

Our understanding of the importance of these foods is also very recent. In the last fifty years, there have been over 10,000 experiments showing the value of consuming high-nutrient plant foods. Here are a few critical points from these studies:

- Plants contain three classes of micronutrients that are critical for our health: vitamins, minerals, and phytochemicals. The finding of thousands of phytochemical compounds in natural plant foods is the most significant discovery in nutritional science in this century. We have learned that these nutrients are essential for a highly effective immune system and protection from the common diseases of aging.

- A plant-based diet that is rich in colorful vegetables and fruits allows you to eat more food. With so many high-nutrient foods permitted in a relatively unlimited quantity, it makes it easy to eat to fulfillment and still lose weight, without the need to count calories or restrict portions.

- Increasing micronutrients and reducing calories enables the body to produce an assortment of protective health benefits and defy the aging process. In essence, these studies have shown that there is a way to extend life and delay the onset of aging, allowing you to live better and to be healthier in your later years.

Fifty years of scientific studies indicate that most diseases seen in modern countries, as well as the leading causes of death, are the result of dietary and lifestyle choices. Scientists have determined that inadequate consumption of plant-derived nutrients results in cellular toxicity, DNA damage, and immune system dysfunction. This, in turn, leads to increased susceptibility to infections, allergies, and even the development of cancer.

There is a way to eat that helps prevent these health problems and satisfies your hunger with fewer calories. A diet rich in high-nutrient plant foods is the most effective way to reduce your food cravings. As your level of micronutrients increases—by consuming greater amounts of high-nutrient foods—your appetite will naturally decrease. The result is that you will become healthier and will look and feel young well into your later years. There is no reason for anyone to develop heart disease, strokes, Type II diabetes, or dementia. To prevent and reverse these and most other chronic diseases, you don't need instructions from a doctor's prescription pad. The prescription is nutrition.

Unhealthful food choices

Many people suffer from medical ailments because they were never taught about their genuine nutritional requirements. As a country, we eat entirely too many low-nutrient foods, which deliver too many calories and not enough nutrients. When our nutrient-deprived bodies then crave more food, the easy availability of calorie-rich, low-nutrient foods enables us to eat ourselves to death. A diet based on milk, meats, cheese, pasta, bread, fried foods, and sugar-filled snacks and drinks lays the groundwork for obesity, cancer, heart disease, diabetes, digestive disorders, and autoimmune illnesses.

Unhealthful foods harmful in three ways

It is important to understand why the foods I just mentioned are harmful.

1) They are high in disease-promoting substances that undermine our health.

2) The more unhealthful foods you eat, the fewer health-promoting, plant-based foods you will eat.

3) Consuming calories that are lacking antioxidant vitamins and phytochemicals leads to a buildup of waste products in your cells because your body can't remove normal cellular wastes without sufficient nutrients. The cells don't have the raw materials needed for optimal or normal function. The lack of some substances and the excess of others ages us prematurely and causes disease.

Foods such as chips, cookies, bread, and pasta lose a dramatic amount of their nutrients during the refinement process. Plus, the process that browns foods and turns a grain into a baked flake or chip creates acrylamides—carcinogens that make these foods even more harmful. In addition to being nutrient-poor, processed foods contain ingredients that contribute to health problems: salt, chemical food additives, trans fats, MSG, sodium nitrate, and other unhealthful ingredients.

By contrast, unrefined plant foods, including vegetables, beans, nuts, seeds, and fruits, are the most nutrient-dense foods. Unfortunately, the average American consumes less than 7 percent of his or her calories from these foods. People who eat according to my guidelines, however, consume 70-90 percent of their calories from unrefined plant foods. By increasing the amount of nutrient-dense food you eat, you are directly influencing your body's chance to thrive.

THE POWER OF MICRONUTRIENTS

All the different types of nutrients are vital to achieving and maintaining optimal health; however, phytochemicals hold a special, elite place in the nutritional landscape. When consistently consumed in sufficient quantities and varieties, phytochemicals become supernutrients in your body. They work together to detoxify cancer-causing compounds, deactivate free radicals, protect against radiation damage, and enable DNA repair mechanisms.[20] When altered or broken strands of DNA are repaired, you are less likely to develop cancer later in life.

Consuming phytochemicals is not optional. They are essential in human immune-system defenses. Without a wide variety and sufficient amount of phytochemicals from unprocessed plant foods, cells age more rapidly and do not retain their innate ability to remove and detoxify waste products and toxic compounds. Low levels of phytochemicals in our modern diet are largely responsible for the common diseases seen with aging, especially cancer and heart disease. These are diseases caused by nutritional ignorance and, in the majority of cases, can be prevented. Approximately 85 percent of our population suffers from and eventually dies of heart disease, strokes, and cancer. This is extremely high compared to other populations around the world and at earlier points in human history.

Let's take heart disease as an example. Heart attacks are extremely rare occurrences in populations that eat a diet rich in protective phytochemicals, such as the Okinawans of Japan, but are omnipresent in populations, such as ours, that eat a diet low in protective nutrients.[21] Compelling data from numerous population and interventional studies shows that a natural, plant-based diet rich in antioxidants and phytochemicals will prevent, arrest, and even reverse heart disease.[22] With what we know about heart disease causation, no one needs to die of heart disease today.

Only via superior nutrition can you attack all the invisible, but potentially dangerous plaque throughout your coronary arteries. Unlike surgery and angioplasty, the dietary approach addressed in this book does not merely treat a small segment of your heart. It rejuvenates all your blood vessels and protects your entire body against heart attacks, strokes, venous thrombosis and pulmonary embolisms, peripheral vascular disease, and vascular dementia.

To receive the benefits of modern nutritional science, however, you must actually eat well. Many people believe that they can meet all of their nutrient needs by taking supplements. However, supplements can't match or duplicate all the protective, strengthening elements of real fruits and vegetables. There are too many unknown and undiscovered factors in these natural foods. There are more than 10,000 identified phytochemicals, with more being discovered all the time. Only by eating a diet rich in whole foods can you provide yourself with a full complement of these disease-protecting, anti-aging nutrients. Supplements can be useful in delivering micronutrients found in foods that would be very difficult to incorporate into our diet, such as the iodine found in seaweed. But keep in mind that supplements, as the word implies, are *supplemental* to a healthful diet, not a replacement for it.

Our bodies were designed to make use of thousands of plant compounds. When these necessary compounds are missing, we might survive because our bodies are adaptable, but we pay a price. Without them, we lose our powerful potential for wellness. Chronic diseases often develop, and we are robbed of living to our fullest potential in good physical, emotional, and mental health. Ultimately, we are what we eat. We get the materials to build our cells from our diet because food provides the raw materials that our bodies use to create tissue and to function at a high level. Consumption of healthful foods leads to disease resistance; consumption of unhealthful foods makes us disease-prone. Eating right enables you to feel your best every day. You may still get sick from a virus, but your body will be in a far better position to defend itself and make a quick and complete recovery. Optimal nutrition enables you to work better, play better, and maintain your youthful vigor as you age gracefully.

Micronutrient density

For optimal health, you need to eat foods that are high in micronutrients per calorie. This important nutritional concept can be presented by a simple mathematical formula, which I call my health equation.

Dr Fuhrman's Health Equation: H = N/C

Your future Health (H) will increase as your Nutrient (N)* to Calorie (C) ratio increases.

* Nutrient (N) refers to *micro*nutrients.

Your health is dependent on the nutrient-per-calorie density of your diet (micronutrients consumed divided by calories consumed). This straightforward mathematical formula is the basis of nutritional science and nutritional healing. For you to build and maintain excellent health, your diet must be micronutrient-rich, and you must not overeat on calories or macronutrients. The nutrient density in your body's tissues is proportional to the nutrient density of your diet. Choose foods and design your diet with this equation in mind. Consume more foods with a high nutrient-per-calorie density and fewer foods with a low nutrient-per-calorie density. Make every calorie count.

How do you know which foods have the highest nutrient-per-calorie density? To answer this question, I have ranked the nutrient density of many common foods in the table below using my *Dr. Fuhrman's Nutrient Density Scores*. These scores rank a variety of foods based on how many nutrients they deliver to your body for each calorie consumed. The highest score that a food can get is 100. Food labels, when they are required at all, list only a few nutrients, but my scores are based on twenty-three important micronutrients. The scores let you quickly see which foods promote the healthiest outcomes. That way, you can evaluate the quality of your current diet and get an idea of how much better it will be when you start adding high-nutrient foods (and eliminating low-nutrient ones). The scores are a simple way to help you identify and eat larger amounts of high-nutrient foods. The higher the scores and the greater percentage of those foods in your diet, the better your health will be. Take a look at the scores. How do the foods you eat rate?

Highest-nutrient foods

Because phytochemicals are largely unnamed and unmeasured, the nutrient-density scores may underestimate the healthful properties of colorful, natural, plant foods compared to processed foods and animal products. One thing we do know about natural foods is this: The foods that contain the highest amount of known nutrients are the same foods that contain the most unknown nutrients. So, even though these scores may need to be revised somewhat as science uncovers new phytochemicals, they still represent a reasonable guide to understanding the value of the foods you eat.

DR. FUHRMAN'S NUTRIENT DENSITY SCORES

Mustard greens	100	Mushrooms	35
Watercress	100	Tomato	33
Kale	100	Pomegranate	30
Turnip greens	100	Carrots	30
Collard greens	100	Blueberries	27
Brussels sprouts	90	Orange	27
Bok choy	85	Grapes	24
Spinach	82	Edamame	21
Arugula	77	Cherries	21
Cabbage	59	Tofu	20
Flaxseed	55	Sesame seeds	19
Broccoli	52	Sunflower seeds	16
Cauliflower	51	Artichoke	16
Romaine	45	Lentils	14
Green bell pepper	41	Cantaloupe	12
Onions	37	Peaches	11
Asparagus	36	Kidney beans	11
Strawberries	35	Walnuts	10

Iceberg lettuce	10	Skim milk	2
Pistachio nuts	9	Low-fat plain yogurt	2
Cucumber	9	Whole wheat bread	2
Sweet potato	9	Olive oil	2
Green peas	7	Apple juice	1
Almonds	7	White bread	1
Pineapple	7	Chicken breast	1
Avocado	6	Eggs	1
Cashews	6	White pasta	1
Apple	5	Shrimp	1
Mango	5	Ground beef, 85% lean	-4
Peanut butter	5	Feta cheese	-5
Corn	4	Low-fat cheddar cheese	-6
Bananas	3	Potato chips	-9
Brown rice	3	French fries	-9
Oatmeal	3	Vanilla ice cream	-9
White potato	2	Cola	-10
Salmon	2		

DR. FUHRMAN'S NUTRIENT DENSITY SCORES

To determine the scores, an equal-calorie serving of each food was evaluated. The following nutrients were included in the evaluation: calcium, carotenoids (beta carotene, alpha carotene, lutein, zeaxanthin, and lycopene), fiber, folate, glucosinolates, magnesium, selenium, vitamin C, vitamin E, zinc, phytosterols, resistant starch, flavonoids, plus ORAC score. ORAC (Oxygen Radical Absorbance Capacity) is a measure of the antioxidant or radical-scavenging capacity of a food. For consistency, nutrient quantities were converted from their typical measurement conventions (mg, mcg, IU) to a percentage of their Reference Daily Intake (RDI). For nutrients that have no RDI, goals were established based on available research and current understanding of the benefits of these factors. Points were added if the food item was anti-angiogenic or contained organosulfides, aromatase inhibitors, or resveratrol. Points were subtracted if the food item contained trans fat, an excessive amount of saturated fat, cholesterol, or sodium, or was a refined or processed food with harmful additives. To make it easier to compare foods, the raw point totals were converted (multiplied by the same number) so that the highest ranking food (mustard greens) received a score of 100, and the other foods received lower scores accordingly.

As expected, green vegetables win the prize, and no other food is even close. No wonder green vegetables have the best association with lower rates of cancer and heart disease. While most people get the majority of their calories from foods with the lower scores, if you increase your consumption of foods with higher scores, you can dramatically improve your health. The recipes and menus in *3 Steps to Incredible Health, Volume 2* will help you achieve this goal.

In any of the levels of the high-nutrient diet, there are some foods that you can eat in relatively unlimited quantities, the ultimate foods in terms of nutrient density and excellence. Memorize the categories below. If you can learn to make your recipes and meals mostly from the foods in the higher categories, you will be maximizing the nutrient density of your diet. You will protect yourself from illness and disease in the future and have the greatest chance of recovering your health if you are currently unhealthy.

High-nutrient foods that can be eaten in nearly unlimited quantities (without overeating, of course):

Leafy green vegetables
romaine lettuce, leaf lettuces, kale, collards, Swiss chard, cabbage, spinach, bok choy, parsley

Solid green vegetables
artichokes, asparagus, broccoli, brussels sprouts, cabbage, celery, cucumber, kohlrabi, okra, peas, green peppers, snow peas, string beans, zucchini

Non-green, high-nutrient vegetables
beets, eggplant, mushrooms, onions, tomatoes, peppers, bamboo shoots, water chestnuts, cauliflower, squash, carrots

Beans and legumes
red kidney beans, adzuki beans, chickpeas, pinto beans, cowpeas, navy beans, cannellini beans, soybeans, lentils, white beans, lima beans, pigeon peas, black-eyed peas, black beans, split peas

Fresh fruits

apples, apricots, blackberries, blueberries, grapes, kiwis, mangoes, nectarines, all melons, oranges, peaches, pears, persimmons, pineapples, plums, raspberries, strawberries, tangerines

BUILDING A BETTER FOOD PYRAMID

By now, you understand that the key to high-level health is eating more vegetables, fruits, and other nutrient-rich foods. Let's divide food into three types: animal products, processed foods, and unprocessed plant foods. The high-nutrient diet dramatically reduces both animal products and processed foods in your diet and increases consumption of unprocessed plant foods, the most nutrient-rich foods on the planet. Even among the unprocessed plant foods, I encourage you to eat more of the most cancer-protective foods, such as greens, mushrooms, and onions.

Over the years, Americans have become accustomed to seeing the United States Department of Agriculture (USDA) food pyramid, which purports to be a guide to healthful food choices. Unfortunately, the design of the food pyramid has always been strongly influenced by social, business, and political concerns, not pure science. As a result, the USDA pyramid is not a reliable guide. This is one reason why so many Americans are confused about nutrition and plagued with obesity and preventable diseases. If you wanted to design a food pyramid that would actually help people, the base would consist of foods that should be consumed in the highest quantity, followed by foods that should be consumed regularly, followed by foods that should be consumed infrequently. The USDA pyramid doesn't do this. In fact, its design encourages people to regularly eat foods that should only be eaten rarely, if at all.

I propose a new pyramid. For superior health, we must eat more nutrient-rich foods and fewer low-nutrient, high-calorie foods. The top of my pyramid is composed of the foods lowest in nutrients, such as processed foods like chips and cookies. These are the foods that should be consumed very rarely, if at all. The base is comprised of the nutrient-rich plant foods according to their nutrient composition and disease-protective properties.

These include:

- green and other low-starch vegetables

- fresh fruits

- beans or legumes

- nuts, seeds, and avocados

- starchy vegetables (mostly root vegetables)

- whole grains

When the nutritional landscape of America is shaped by nutrient density as represented in the pyramid below, we will have dramatically extended our population's healthy life expectancy, and we will see health care costs plummet.

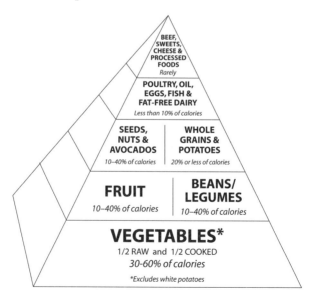

Dangers of omission

Our society has evolved to a level of economic sophistication that allows us to eat ourselves to death. A diet centered on milk, cheese, pasta, bread, fried foods, and sugar-filled snacks and drinks lays the groundwork for obesity, cancer, heart disease, diabetes, and autoimmune illnesses. These foods certainly are harmful, but that is not the whole problem. Part of the problem is that we are not eating enough nutrient-rich foods.

America's Food Consumption Pie

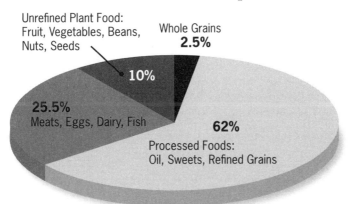

United States Department of Agriculture Economics Research Service, 2005.
http://www.ers.usda.gov/Data/FoodConsumption/FoodGuideIndex.htm#calories

As this chart shows, when you evaluate the standard American diet (SAD), you find that the calories coming from phytochemical-rich foods, such as fresh fruit, vegetables, beans, raw nuts, and seeds, are less than 13 percent of the total caloric intake. This dangerously low intake of unrefined plant foods guarantees weakened immunity to disease, frequent illnesses, and a shorter life span. We will never win the war on cancer, heart disease, diabetes, autoimmune diseases, and other degenerative illnesses until we address this deficiency. The American diet has spread all over the world, taking with it heart disease, cancer, and obesity, but studies still show that in the populations that eat more fruits and vegetables, the incidences of death from these diseases is dramatically lower.[23]

Most health authorities today are in agreement that we should add more servings of fruits and vegetables to our diet. I disagree somewhat. Thinking about our diet in this fashion doesn't adequately address the problem. Instead of thinking of adding the protective fruits, vegetables, beans, and nuts to a disease-causing diet, these foods must be the main focus of the diet. This is what makes my high-nutrient approach different. Once we make nutrient-rich vegetables, fruits, beans, and nuts the caloric foundation of the diet, then maybe we can safely add a few small servings of lower-nutrient foods like animal products and grains.

Foods to die for

Most Americans are not in good health, thanks to the standard, low-nutrient diet in this country. The risk of developing high blood pressure, diabetes, and heart disease or dying prematurely from cardiovascular-related disease is extremely high for all people who eat this way. Look at these statistics:

- The lifetime risk for developing hypertension (high blood pressure) is over 90 percent.[24]

- High blood pressure has climbed 30 percent over the past decade.

- Cardiovascular disease (CVD) is an enormous health care burden and is responsible for approximately 40 percent of all U.S. deaths annually.[25]

There's nothing preprogrammed in the human genome that says as people get old they automatically get fat and have high blood pressure. They develop high blood pressure because their diets are calorie-rich and nutrient-poor. High blood pressure and heart disease are not the consequences of aging. They are the result of slow insidious damage created from years and years of poor dietary choices.

Processed foods, too much salt, and lack of physical exercise all contribute to the problem. Then people are given prescription drugs that allow them to continue their disease-causing habits while gaining a false sense of security. If you eat like other Americans, you will either have a heart attack and die when you are young, or you will inevitably develop high blood pressure and then be at high risk for either a heart attack or stroke when you get older. Populations around the world who live and eat a more wholesome, plant-based diet have elderly members who are free of high blood pressure.[26] These diseases have known nutritional causes, and you never need to suffer from them.

Today, two in five Americans are obese, and the three out of five Americans who are not obese are significantly overweight. We are in worse shape today, with heavier bodies and thicker waistlines, than at any time in human history. At the same time, scientists have learned that our waistlines and our weight are the most critical factors governing our health and life span. In spite of an overwhelming amount of scientific evidence showing that we could prevent it, people still are dying prematurely and living poor quality lives plagued by sickness and disability. Heart disease, diabetes, and most cancers are preventable, but prevention requires change. It sounds simple, and it can be simple if you have an open mind and if you let knowledge, rather than habits and emotions, guide you.

Learn from your elders

Our bodies are designed to live long and healthy lives, free from the common diseases of aging. However, years of abuse leaves its toll. If water runs over a waterfall and pounds into a rock at high speed, it wears down and eventually splits the rock in two. It was not aging that broke the rock; it was the water that took its toll on it after many thousands of years. Likewise, we develop hardening of the arteries, high blood pressure, heart disease, dementia, and other debilitating conditions from our dietary follies that take their toll over many years of nutritional self-abuse. These common ailments are not the consequence of aging. They are earned.

Researchers have found that people who exceed 100 years of age can be remarkably disease-free. Boston and Harvard scientists recording the New England Centenarian Study (NECS) have been studying many long-lived individuals. Among other factors, they tracked genetics, physical and mental health, and lifestyle habits. They found that long-lived people generally do not have the age-associated medical conditions that develop and curtail enjoyment of life at an early age. In other words, living healthfully goes hand in hand with living longer. These people, who are now past 100, did not have the advantage of the scientific information that we have today. For the majority of their lives, they did not have access to the healthiest foods. The question is, how did they do it, and what skills can we learn from these super seniors?

For starters, none of these centenarians were overweight. To achieve your maximum health potential, you must manage your weight. You can literally stretch your life span by shrinking your waistline. Developing a healthful diet and maintaining a stable, lower weight is the most powerful anti-aging weapon in your arsenal. However, we also must consider evidence that nutritional deficiencies have been shown to cause disease and disability. The goal is to maintain a high or adequate nutrient intake and ensure that no deficiencies exist, while making sure we do not consume excess calories. Yet again, the secret is incorporating large amounts of high-nutrient, low-calorie foods into your diet.

When looking at long-lived, elderly people within a society like ours, in which people eat similarly and the average age of death is about seventy-five, we are selecting individuals with favorable genetics. Scientific studies don't tell us much because most of our population eats the standard (disease-causing) diet, so when we look at outcomes, they merely reflect genetic influences, not vast differences in the consumption of micronutrients. It would be more revealing if we could look at an entire population that has an average life span over the age of ninety and see what the population did to achieve that accomplishment. John Robbins' book, *Healthy At 100,* reviewed the lifestyles of the longest-lived populations around the globe in recent world history. The top three societies were the Abkhasia in the Caucasus south of Russia, the Vilcabamba in the Andes of South America, and the Hunza in Central Asia. These isolated cultures not only experience a population with very long average lives, but their elderly also experience excellent health, free of common diseases seen in our modern world.

The diets in all of these ultra long-lived societies contain at least 90 percent of calories from unrefined foods: high-nutrient fruits, vegetables, beans, nuts, and seeds. Animal products are a much smaller part of the diet, ranging from 1-10 percent of calories. These societies consist of physically active people who grow most of their own food and eat mostly fresh vegetables and fruits. The longest lived societies on record all follow a high-nutrient diet. These healthy societies reveal that, in addition to being slim, there are other important factors that super-seniors share.

- They consume the majority of calories from fresh produce.

- They have an optimistic outlook on life.

- They maintain a social circle of friends.

- They stay physically active.

Analyzing the results of these studies in terms of diet, it seems clear that a dietary program that will enable dramatic increases in life span and protection against later-life diseases includes high-nutrient foods and excludes excess calories and nutrient deficiencies.

The more nutrients, especially antioxidants and phytochemicals, that you consume, and the more variety of each consumed, the better immune function and resistance to disease you achieve. You can see these benefits at any age. I have elderly patients who have been coming to see me for more than ten years, and I have seen their blood-pressure and cholesterol readings fall gradually over the ten-year period while they were following my dietary suggestions. Rather than seeing the gradual rise in blood pressure and cholesterol with age, I have observed the opposite. After many years, they eventually reach the low systolic blood pressures we commonly see in children. The point is that aging is not the cause of your rise in blood pressure; it is the time spent eating the conventional American diet that takes its toll.

To increase your chances of becoming one of these super seniors, you should eat lots of whole foods that are naturally rich in protective nutrients. Take advantage of the fresh produce shipped all over the country. Never before in human history has year-round access to such high-quality food been available to such a large population. Eating high-nutrient foods will make it very likely that more people can survive into their hundreds and live healthier than ever before. Even if your genetic potential does not match most of these super-seniors, you can still have the opportunity for a long, healthy life because you can choose to eat high on the nutrient-density line. Nutrition and other lifestyle factors that you choose are more significant determinants of your health than genetics.

Virtually all disease is the result of the interaction of genetics and modifiable environmental and behavioral factors. Rarely does a single gene variant lead to the development of disease. Common diseases such as cancer, heart disease, and diabetes result from the complex interplay of genes and environment and cannot be classified as only genetic or environmental. The reality is that both genetics and the environment contribute to disease, and the biggest component of environmental causation is diet.

A good example is breast cancer. Less than 1 percent of women living in rural China get breast cancer, whereas 18 percent of American women eventually suffer with the disease. Yet when Asian women immigrate to America and adopt the richer American diet, which is higher in calories and animal products and lower in vegetables, they suffer the same breast cancer rates as other Americans.[27] Genes interact with environmental factors to influence an individual's susceptibility to disease. When these environmental promoters are not present, the disease simply does not appear.

Despite medical advances, 85 percent of Americans still will die from heart disease, cancer, or diabetes. The real key to longevity is not better treatment; it is prevention. In comparison with our sickly nation, people who survive past 100 years are remarkably disease-free. They are generally physically active, independent, and socially connected. They are not the feeble stereotypes that we often associate with getting old. This is not merely about living longer; it is also about staying younger and healthier into your later years, so life can be enjoyed to its fullest. Once you grasp the possibilities, your entire way of thinking will change. You do not have to be a victim. You can experience a long, disease-free life!

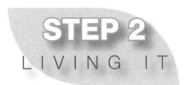

STEP 2
LIVING IT

FOOD ADDICTIONS
AND THE DESIRE TO OVEREAT

Before we take *Step 2* and start learning about Food Addictions and the Desire to Overeat, here are some more success stories. One of the things that I find remarkable is that people who come to my office or read my books trying to find a solution to a particular problem end up solving all of their other problems at the same time. That is part of the power and predictability of superior nutrition. As you eat and live in the proper way to maximize your health, your body makes all kinds of positive changes.

As you read through the next few success stories, think about how much healthier and happier you are going to be once you make my high-nutrient program a regular and permanent part of your life. You may wonder if your particular problems can be solved, but almost all problems come from the same source—unhealthful living. Start living right, and you will be amazed at what can happen.

JENNIE — MIGRAINES AND ALLERGIES

I am a twenty-six-year-old mother of one, a military wife, and a home-maker. Since childhood, I've had an issue with my weight, self-image, eating habits, and energy levels. I was always fatigued and regularly woke up more exhausted than when I went to bed. Over time, my allergies and activity-induced asthma became worse. I felt like a shell of a person. I was disgusted with myself for being so unhealthy at my young age. My life was out of control, and I felt helpless. One minute, I would have the strength to eat healthfully, and the next minute I would cave in and eat junk food. The food addiction set me up for a ritualistic "try and fail" dance that chipped away at my self-esteem.

In my early twenties, I took a laundry list of prescriptions for depression, migraine headaches, and allergies (requiring an inhaler and two allergy shots per week). I had a drug to wake me up in the morning and one to put me to sleep at night. I had the resumé of a hypochondriac, only I wasn't one. Western medicine just kept throwing drugs my way instead of looking for the causes of the ailments.

Doctors had me believing that "these things just happen" for no apparent reason. They expected me to take drugs for the rest of my life.

After I had my son, I began seeking a different path. Thankfully, I discovered Dr. Fuhrman's *Eat to Live*. That book inspired me and helped me lose 43 pounds in five months (from 158 to 115 pounds), and I am now off all medications except for one that I use infrequently for allergies. I have no migraines, acne, or depression. Best of all, the sleep disorder has completely vanished!

I'm jubilant now that I'm in control of my life! I'm in the driver's seat instead of being the victim of food cravings. My skin glows instead of being plagued with blemishes. I go out more, because I don't have to try on fifty different outfits trying not to look fat. You wouldn't think a high-nutrient diet could change a person's state of mind, but I've changed from being sad, angry, and wishing I were somebody else, to loving myself. I feel alive. I'm in tune with my body now, and I feel like I've been born into a whole new life that's full of possibilities!

RON — OBESITY AND HEART DISEASE

For someone who considered himself an athlete, I was in bad shape. I had low energy, constant bloating, continual food cravings, and trouble breathing when trying to run a few miles and also when trying to sleep at night. The results of my annual physical were terrible. In addition to being obese (215 pounds), my cholesterol had risen to 231. My doctor wanted me to start taking Lipitor, but I was not excited about putting a drug into my body that would have negative side effects. I wondered if there was a way I could avoid it. If these worries weren't enough, I could not get a new life insurance policy.

Fortunately, I found out about Dr. Fuhrman and started following his program. After just eight weeks, my energy level is higher than ever, the bloating and food cravings are gone, and my breathing is fine. My overall cholesterol dropped from 231 to 127, my LDL cholesterol dropped from 168 to 82, my triglycerides dropped from 142 to 56, and I've lost more than 40 pounds. I've qualified for the highest level of life insurance at the lowest premium rate, and I just completed my first marathon!

DORIS — DIABETES, HIGH BLOOD PRESSURE, AND HIGH CHOLESTEROL

My husband, who was quite overweight, was diagnosed with diabetes. His blood sugar and cholesterol were extremely high. His A1C hemoglobin was 12.7. The doctor gave him no dietary recommendations and simply referred him to a specialist. My husband decided to research diabetes on the Internet, and he discovered Dr. Fuhrman's high-nutrient program. He followed it exactly, and by the time he saw the specialist four weeks later, his blood results were normal. They remain normal, as do his follow-up blood exams. He has lost 65 pounds. If I hadn't seen this with my own eyes, I would not believe it.

TED — TYPE I DIABETES AND WEIGHT LOSS

I have had Type I diabetes for twenty-five years and have been on many different regimes, including an insulin pump. But prior to following Dr. Fuhrman's recommendations, never had I seen my blood sugars so good. I am working toward my target weight and feeling better all the time. I heartily encourage all Type I diabetics to try this program. It could save your life. But do consider working with a physician because the need for insulin can drop quickly, and it is important that it be monitored. So far, I am down 30 percent on my insulin dose, which is quite unusual for a Type I diabetic. I am stunned!

ROSITA — WEIGHT LOSS

I was thin as a child, but once I got to college I began eating more and more convenience foods and prepackaged meals. By the time I gave birth to my second son, I was carrying 50 extra pounds. I tried to research the best way to eat, but the information was contradictory and confusing. I drank diet drinks and ate low-fat dairy products, skinless chicken breast and turkey, and nonfat dressings, but my weight climbed steadily. At the age of thirty-eight, I tipped the scales at 210 pounds. I thought something had to be wrong with my metabolism, and I was ready to give up and accept that obesity was my fate in life.

Dr. Fuhrman's message opened my eyes to a new way of thinking about food and hunger. His book helped me understand why all the low-fat meats and grains fed my drive to overeat, and why I was always fighting off a constant desire to consume more food. I started following his advice to eat for high-nutrient density, and the first week I lost 11 pounds. Plus, I wasn't hungry anymore. The new way of eating was a bit of an adjustment at first, but the results were so quick and amazing that I was motivated to push through it. I actually ate more food than I had been eating, but the more I ate, the more weight I lost. I think all the extra nutrients were helping my body rid itself of excess fat. Eight months later, my headaches were gone.

I no longer feel hungry between meals, and I rarely have food cravings (and when I do, it's for leafy greens). I am enjoying my healthful meals, and I feel so much better. I have the energy to exercise again—and enjoy it. Not only do I feel better, but my hair, skin, and nails are in the best shape ever. Oh, by the way, I'm 65 pounds lighter!

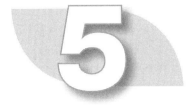

EXERCISES WITH FOOD: THE WARM-UP

Now that you understand the basic principles of the high-nutrient diet, it's time to take *Step 2* and learn about Food Addictions and the Desire to Overeat. Let's start putting some of the principles that you have learned into practice. This chapter features some dietary exercises to help you get started. It is important that you think of these exercises in the same way that you think of exercises at the gym. When you go to the gym, you don't expect to suddenly build muscle; that takes time. You may not even enjoy going to the gym when you first start out. The enjoyment comes later, when you see your body starting to change.

You can apply this same way of thinking to your new way of eating. The dietary exercises that follow will begin to increase your appreciation of natural whole foods. The foods may seem foreign at first, and you may not experience the same enjoyment that you are accustomed to. But that is to be expected. As with exercise, the enjoyment comes later, when you start to enjoy your new meals and start to see your body changing. The exercises expose your palate to new sensations, which can take time to get used to. Some people mistakenly conclude that the food will never taste good. A better way of thinking about it is that the tastes and textures are *unfamiliar,* and that they will take a little time to get used to. That is why I designed these exercises. Start small, and progress at your own speed. Don't do too much too fast, but do your exercises consistently.

EXERCISE 1

The first exercise is to eat one-half pound of cut up raw vegetables and one-half pound of low-calorie fruits each day. This is not that much food. You should do this exercise at the same time each day. I recommend eating the fruit at breakfast and the raw vegetables in the afternoon before dinner. The important thing is to do the exercise close to mealtime and not when you have a full stomach. You should feel like eating. Remember not to eat too heavily at lunch, so that you are hungry enough later in the afternoon, before dinner, to eat your extra raw vegetables. The goal of this exercise is to eat a comfortable amount of raw vegetables, including tomatoes, red pepper, carrots, broccoli spears, celery, snow pea pods, and zucchini, and fruits including fresh berries, cantaloupe, kiwi, and apple slices. Over time, see if you can comfortably increase the volume of food.

After eating all these raw vegetables and fruits, you may decide to eat less at dinner because you feel too full, but let that decision come naturally. Try not to overeat, but don't try to restrict yourself, either. Eat the amount that feels comfortable, and try to stop eating before you feel full. Stop when you're satisfied. Finding the difference between satisfied and full is an important step in becoming a healthy eater.

EXERCISE 2

The second exercise can be done at the same time as the first. While you are eating those fruits and vegetables during the day, chew each mouthful until every piece of food is liquefied. This will take a considerable amount of time and will feel very different from how you are used to eating, but how you eat is very important. Eating slowly is the only way to gain all the nutrients that you want from the food. You can access the full nutrient load from the food by breaking open every single plant cell. Eating this way also will exercise your jaw and help you develop healthier gums and teeth. Remember: Chew, chew, and chew.

The most important element of these exercises is performing them every single day. Doing them daily will not only increase your enjoyment of healthful foods, but also will help you lose weight. In the beginning, you may continue eating some foods from your traditional diet, although you will probably be eating a lot less of them. Over time, you will be more comfortable eliminating your unhealthful food choices and replacing them with healthful ones because your palate will desire them. Let this process happen at its own pace. Do not do these exercises instead of eating a meal, especially in this beginning stage.

A skill is a developed talent or ability, and being healthy is the result of several skills. The difficulty comes when you try to be proficient in all of those skills at once. Enjoying the taste of healthful food is a skill. Giving up old foods that you love in favor of new foods that you don't like requires multiple skills: abstinence and tolerance. These exercises isolate and target specific skill sets. They will help you avoid the anxiety that many feel when they give up their old way of eating all of a sudden. The method that I have developed is a purposeful and effective way to assist you in your transition to preferring a healthful approach to eating.

Warm-up goals

- Have at least three fresh fruits with your breakfast.

- Eat a large salad or raw vegetables as part of your dinner every night, and chew thoroughly.

Some people can jump right in and immediately switch to the ideal, high-nutrient way of eating. I consider the ideal version of this diet to be one that contains at least 90 percent of calories from the most healthful foods: vegetables, fruits, beans, raw nuts and seeds, avocados, and whole grains. For some people, this amount of change might feel too dramatic. It isn't always easy to give up foods that you love and to replace them with unfamiliar ones. Also, some people experience uncomfortable physical or mental symptoms when making the change. The modified approach that you are learning here works in sync with your brain so that you won't feel withdrawal or deprivation.

Don't be afraid to eat healthful foods. The focus here is on eating more, not less. The more raw and cooked green vegetables you consume, the less space you will have to eat high-calorie, low-nutrient foods. As the illustration below demonstrates, you will fill a sizeable volume of space in your stomach with a very small number of calories. This will help you comfortably cut the number of calories that you eat each day. This is very much like gastric bypass surgery without the surgery.

400 CALORIES

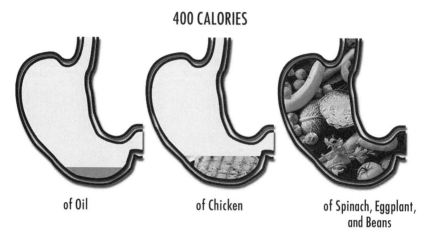

of Oil   of Chicken   of Spinach, Eggplant, and Beans

Adjust the amount of raw vegetables you eat to what your body will comfortably tolerate. If you experience uncomfortable gas, cut back a little on raw vegetables and beans. Don't remove these foods, just cut back partially, because the goal is to let your body adjust the timing and secretion of its digestive enzymes and peristalsis to accommodate this healthful, more natural diet. You should be able to increase the amount of raw vegetables gradually without a problem. Don't forget to concentrate on chewing better because that may solve the problem. It can take time for your digestive system to build up the capacity to digest raw, whole foods, especially if you have been eating a low-fiber diet for a long time.

There is another benefit to chewing well. Eating too quickly encourages overeating and can tax the digestive system. It takes about fifteen minutes for your brain to realize that your stomach is full. If you eat too fast, your body won't have enough time to tell you when it's full. You will end up eating more than you really needed. Slow down, thoroughly chew your food, and enjoy the experience of eating.

THINKING STRAIGHT ABOUT FOOD

It is a sad fact that what we hear about nutrition and dieting from TV, radio, newspapers, diet books, and even most of the scientific research community is thoroughly confusing. Almost every article or show on the topic discusses some magic food, supplement, metabolism booster, or fat-carbohydrate-protein ratio that can solve all of your weight problems. Research articles continue to test diets that are low in fat, high in fat, low in carbohydrates, and high in carbohydrates, and the media is content to report on them as though they represented some important new information about the successes and failures of these various diets. But trying to micromanage carbohydrate, fat, or protein intake will not increase your health or longevity. This sort of dieting only encourages temporary fluctuations in calorie intake, leading to non-sustained changes in body weight, often called yo-yo dieting. These diets are bad for your health because it is not healthful to lose and gain weight over and over. What these studies actually show is that diets that don't address nutrient *quality* do not work.

There is no magical ratio of fat, carbohydrate, or protein that will lead you to your ideal weight and superior health. Rather, science has shown that only substantive changes in the quality of the nutrients you eat (with special attention given to micronutrients) can positively influence your body in terms of health, caloric drive, and weight. You need to learn and adopt a new way of living that will improve your quality of life for years to come. The knowledge is available to maximize nutrition to the point where genetic predispositions will not have the chance to express themselves.

The incredible increase in overweight individuals, obesity, diabetes, and heart disease in the last century did not occur because people changed their genes. It occurred because they changed their diets. The toxic food environment that pervades every city and town can make it difficult for people to find or accept the path back to healthful eating. However, by reading this book and practicing what it preaches, you are setting yourself apart. You are beginning to create a new environment for yourself that allows your body to thrive and maximize its genetic potential, enhancing its disease-protective capacity. If everyone would create that environment for themselves, we would achieve dramatic increases in healthy life expectancy and longevity.

Unlike trendy diets that focused on one or another aspect of food, the high-nutrient diet requires that you use your mind to evaluate all aspects of your approach to food. To be successful in designing a healthful diet for yourself, you must accomplish the following:

1. Reprogram your thinking and tastes to prefer micronutrient-rich foods.

2. Eliminate addictive hunger symptoms that lead to overeating by making micronutrient-rich foods the foundation of your diet.

3. Limit unhealthful foods from your daily diet.

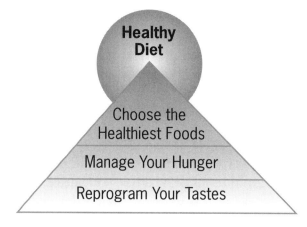

As you increase your intake of high-nutrient food, you will desire unhealthful, low-nutrient food less and less. As you progress through this book, you will continue to limit your intake of such foods, including animal products, saturated fat, and processed foods such as white flour and sugar. In the next chapters, we will discuss managing your hunger and ensuring that you don't overconsume calories. We will focus on how you think about food and how you can reprogram your tastes.

While it is important to understand and think about each of these steps, it's also important to realize that they do not exist independently. We need to eat less fat, protein, and carbohydrates, the only three sources of calories in food. Obviously, we need calories, but we want to make sure that when we do consume them, the fat, protein, and carbohydrates that we choose to eat are in foods that are as micronutrient-dense as possible. The healthiest way to eat—and the way to learn to naturally and automatically desire fewer calories—is to consistently consume high-nutrient meals. When you understand and try to follow all three steps, you will be amazed at how easy and simple it is to achieve your ideal weight and health.

Your powerful mind

My book, *Eat To Live*, was written to help overweight people recover health and lose the stubborn, excess weight by following the most healthful and most effective diet. It was not written for the masses, and has limitations for wide acceptance because people's addictive relationships with unhealthful foods are too overwhelming. For many people, the *Eat To Live* approach was too great a change to implement all at once.

The high-nutrient diet features the same principles, but you will be approaching it in three steps and you will learn about three levels of healthful eating. Many people need to make dramatic changes in the way they think before they can be asked to change the way they eat. They also need to approach the changes gradually, versus all at once. The three levels presented here give you the opportunity to make the changes more gradually. We are all born with an innate desire to not only survive, but to thrive. Somewhere along the line, we have forgotten that fundamental imperative and have picked up so many bad habits that it can take some time to adjust.

In our modern society, we have lost touch with instincts that lead us into healthful, life-sustaining behaviors. We graduate from elementary school, high school, college, and even graduate school and don't learn the one most important thing we should know: how to protect our future health. Consider that 38 percent of our population dies of heart disease and strokes. That number is a deeper tragedy because these are needless and avoidable deaths. The solution is readily available, but few are aware of it.

For many, even when the information is presented to them, the fear of change and of loss of pleasure forces them to close their eyes to it. In a perfect world, all people would live healthfully, get enough sleep, exercise, and eat the high-nutrient diet that would best protect their precious health. Nowadays, this seems almost impossible to do because most people believe that the change would be too hard. For them, my approach seems counterintuitive. It is radically different from what they are used to, and they think it would be too difficult to follow, so they dismiss it. The mountain of supporting scientific evidence is not sufficiently persuasive. They need something more than just cold science to inspire them. Some people are so addicted to their present, dangerous diet that they would prefer death to change. My goal is to uncover and address all the conscious and subconscious impediments you might face.

Conflicting messages

The principal reason why people have difficulty adopting a healthful diet is because they have internal conflict. One part of them wants to be healthy, while another wants to do something that is not healthful, usually something that gives them pleasure in the moment, like eating a pint of ice cream. While you hold the carton and spoon in your hands, you want to eat the ice cream. In the larger perspective, you want to be healthy and lead a long, productive life. You can learn how to rectify these two desires.

Adopting a healthful lifestyle generally requires change on many levels. Each level is controlled by a different region of the brain, and each level is like a different frequency or radio channel. As a result, you need to work on all aspects of yourself until being healthy and maintaining an ideal weight comes naturally. My goal is to help you adopt a healthy set of core beliefs and healthy automatic responses so that eventually you will follow a healthful lifestyle without any conscious effort. The process is not about strengthening your willpower, calorie-counting, or any other gimmick.

To achieve permanent success in the health and weight loss arena, we have to consider the complexity of human nature. We are physical, emotional, and social beings. We must consider all of these factors. If we don't, it increases the chance that we will reject health-giving information as too difficult, in spite of our interest in it. This is a physical manifestation of a subconscious process. Our brains are designed to dim awareness to information that causes us anxiety.

For most people, the idea of overhauling the way they think about food and the way they eat is a source of anxiety. Plus, unhealthful foods are a slow-working poison. Many ailments related to the foods people eat take years to develop, and the only visible issue for most people is their excess weight. Studies have shown that most overweight people routinely underestimate the extent of their obesity and do not see themselves as that overweight. Consequently, it is not too difficult to imagine how so many people can ignore the evidence. They don't see what it has to do with them. This is especially true for people who have low self-esteem.

Addressing your self-worth

The objections of those unwilling to change their diet sometimes have very little to do with food. It is often the direct result of low self-esteem, which makes them vulnerable to negative peer pressure, addictions, and emotional overeating. Some may fear appearing different from others, and they think that changing the way they eat will result in a loss of social status. This is a subconscious perception, but some people are unknowingly governed by it. Others overeat to raise dopamine production in the brain, so that they can dull the frustration and pain of life.

As social animals, our brains require certain hormones that are released when we have positive social interaction. Eliminate these interactions, and the brain will seek out other ways to produce the hormones and receive stimulatory input. This is why people with strong social ties are far less likely to be drawn into compulsive over-eating and other addictive behaviors. Several studies have shown that overeating, like drug and alcohol abuse, leads to dopamine stimulation. For people who are dependent on dopamine surges and who lack the emotional fulfillment that life can provide, consumption of high-calorie foods gives the brain the surge it is looking for. Therefore, they are more compelled to engage in stimulating or toxic eating behavior. Their beliefs about themselves set in motion a chain of chemical events that predisposes them to addictive behaviors. This can make it more difficult to adopt a healthful lifestyle, so it is crucial to identify this and address it to successfully change eating behaviors.

People with low self-esteem do not realize that they are living out a self-fulfilling prophecy. The belief that they are unworthy of attention makes it a reality. We are wired to operate in accordance with our beliefs, and it all happens outside of our awareness. People who believe that they are unworthy tend to shy away from other people and develop habits that further lower their attractiveness to others, ultimately reinforcing their negative beliefs and practices. In doing so, such people often lower their self-perceived social status.

Status is an important factor that affects every facet of your life, including the way that you eat. Although people think it has to do with class, economics, or education, it actually comes from something much deeper than that. It comes from a combination of what people believe about themselves and—most importantly for this discussion— what they believe others believe about them. In short, it is a measure of social acceptance. Lower-status people instinctively look to higher-status people for direction, without being aware of it. Lower-status individuals constantly seek acceptance through compliant behaviors, including eating, drinking, smoking, or taking drugs.

Our self-esteem is a core belief; it deeply affects our behaviors in ways that we only barely perceive. Most of us are unable to judge our own status. To get an accurate measurement, we need to examine our automatic behaviors, the things we do without thinking. What are the principal indicators of low status and low self-esteem? A partial list of these includes:

- conformity or compliance, especially with unhealthful behaviors; a fear of being different

- social shyness or fear of displeasing others

- lowered ability to communicate

- physical aggressiveness

- involvement in dysfunctional family relationships

We need to ask ourselves a series of questions to determine if we are allowing self-degradation to hurt our potential for healthful behaviors that will lead to success and happiness.

- Am I engaged in behaviors that are detrimental to me?

- What are the forces pressuring me to adopt or maintain this behavior?

- Does this behavior increase or diminish my status and self-esteem?

- Am I a trendsetter or a trend-follower?

- Am I avoiding a useful behavior because I don't want others to think I am different?

We need to be able to view ourselves in a favorable light and cultivate behaviors and activities that build pride in ourselves in order to challenge these issues. That pride could come from helping others, being understanding of others, having interests that engage us, developing new skills, and appreciating value and goodness wherever we see it.

List a few reasons you have to be proud of yourself.

_____

_____

_____

_____

_____

_____

Write three things you could do to expand the width or depth of your interests.

_____

_____

_____

_____

_____

_____

These written exercises may not seem to be directly tied to your desire to lose weight and increase your health. However, based on years of working with thousands of patients, I assure you that for many people they are. The key to change is learning social skills so you do not look for bad dietary habits to solve your social problems. Behaviors that lead to poor health lower your emotional well-being and further this cycle. Your beliefs and your diet work hand in hand. Self-confidence is important to your health and dietary choices. If you believe that what you say is worthwhile and attractive to others, this attitude will be transferred to everyone around you, regardless of how you might actually look. When you have a legitimate reason to believe in yourself, you will care for yourself better and be more inclined to eat right.

We are all prone to follow the direction of the group, and most Americans follow a diet that is popular and unhealthful. Does following the crowd give you an excuse to resist change? It is a factor for some people. They want to fit in and will be uncomfortable eating differently because they believe they will be rejected by their reference group. This perceived loss of status from being different can create a subconscious resistance, presenting another obstacle to change. This is an irrational response; following the crowd does not lead to enhanced status or self-respect. Quite the opposite; doing what you think is right will increase your self-esteem and emotional well-being. It is unfortunate that an unhealthful lifestyle and a disease-causing diet gains some psychological advantage as it certainly is more popular. But remember, you can lead the crowd; you can change things around for your social circle. By your example, you not only may save your own life, but you also may save someone else's life that you really care about.

Knowing that you have a group of friends who help you to be a better person and with whom you have something in common raises your emotional health and self-confidence. It is far easier to change and transition into a healthful lifestyle when you have the support of others doing the same. The more your group embraces and supports you in your efforts to eat healthier and live a health-supporting lifestyle, the easier this becomes. Our American reference group is a nation eating itself to death, committing suicide with their knives and forks. Given that, it is helpful to have support when attempting to move away from the dietary norm. If you have a real and tangible like-minded social group, you are much less likely to be affected by the artificial ones created by advertisers, marketers, and technology. If you want to get healthy, hang around other healthy people and others striving to be healthy.

Some people will attempt to make you uncomfortable because you are eating healthfully. Your change in behavior may make them uncomfortable because you are forcing them to examine their own unhealthful practices. If you look for approval from someone who is struggling with that issue, you generally will not get a positive response. Don't let people with unhealthful and self-destructive food habits influence your food choices. Control your health destiny. Don't let the reaction of others subconsciously prevent you from adopting this program. Regardless of the illogical motives of the unconscious mind to save face, you actually lower your social status by letting these forces govern your life's choices.

Eating healthfully and developing the skills to earn and enjoy excellent health will contribute to your self-esteem, which in turn will help you socially. This is very important as we know from looking at the data on centenarians in Chapter 4. The *Australian Longitudinal Study of Aging* showed that people with good relationships were 22 percent less likely to die over the following decade.[28] Interestingly, close contact with children and relatives had little impact on survival. It was those with the strongest network of friends and acquaintances who were the most likely to survive. Unquestionably, developing peers who are also interested in healthful living is a great idea. Forming a support group or even joining our online support group (www. DrFuhrman.com) can be extremely beneficial and aid in your success.

Knowledge the key

Even if you have fine self-esteem and a supportive group of people around you, your mind can hold you back from reaching the goals you have for your body. We most often behave in a manner consistent with the way we think. Some of the principles that you are learning as part of this style of eating may seem counterintuitive at first because they do not fit neatly into your prior beliefs. Because we are social animals, ideas seem more believable when more people believe them. They require social proof before they gain general acceptance.

A study published in the *European Journal of Clinical Nutrition* looked at some of the factors that inhibit people from adopting a healthier, plant-based diet. The study found that the more knowledge subjects obtained about the benefits, the more they had their questions answered, and the more prior myths were shattered with science, then the more likely they were to adapt to a healthful diet and achieve good health.[29] For some, change needs to occur in steps, and it has to be at their own pace. Remember, however, that your willingness to change and your success is proportional to the knowledge you obtain. Gaining the knowledge is the most critical factor to enable behavioral changes that will lead to healthier habits.

Some people will decide to ignore the life-enhancing information presented here. That decision often is made on a subconscious level. Unfortunately, the subconscious mind is not logical. A multitude of diets, nutritional supplements, and even drugs promise weight loss without changing the way you eat. These promises give the subconscious mind a way out, an excuse to do nothing, and often are enough to dissuade people from even considering change.

Many of these diets have been debunked, but that doesn't damage their allure to our subconscious minds where most decisions are made. The good news is that you are not at the mercy of your genes or your subconscious mind. You can control your health and weight. Heart diseases, strokes, cancer, dementia, diabetes, allergies, arthritis, and other common illnesses are not predominantly genetic. They are the result of incorrect dietary choices. With knowledge, you will be empowered to make new choices by changing the way that you think.

Ideas have a life of their own. Once they are accepted and popular, they become difficult to displace. Much of what is now widely accepted as nutritional gospel is based on scant evidence, mistaken old notions, bad science, and myths advertised to us by food manufacturers, pharmaceutical companies, supplement marketers, and the government. These myths are so pervasive that even most scientists and physicians accept them. Many current, popular dietary notions have uncertain origins, but since they have been around a long time, they generally go unquestioned. Once they become this ingrained, they are difficult to change, and they form our cognitive health model. When people are presented with new information that falls outside the model, it is difficult to accept.

Here are some commonly held nutritional myths. See if you can figure out whether they are true or false.

Frequent small meals aid weight control. **FALSE**

Frequent eating has been shown to increase calorie consumption. In addition, scientific studies have shown that *reduced* meal frequency increases the life span of both rodents and monkeys, even when the calories consumed were the same in the group fed more frequently and the group fed less frequently.[30] The body needs time between meals to complete digestion. Only when digestion process has ended can the body most effectively detoxify and promote cellular repair. To maximize health, it is not favorable to be constantly eating and digesting food.

Being overweight is due to poor genetics. **FALSE**

Genetics play a role in obesity, and people whose parents are obese have a tenfold increased risk of being obese. However, there are many people with obese parents who are slender and healthy. It is the combination of food choices, inactivity, and genetics that determines the likelihood of obesity.[31] Excellent nutrition and a healthy lifestyle will overwhelm genetics and allow even those with a genetic hindrance to achieve a healthy weight.

Milk builds and strengthens bones. **FALSE**

Medical studies confirm that drinking cow's milk does not lead to stronger bones. In a comprehensive review of all studies of dairy intake and bone strength in 2000, researchers concluded, "The body of scientific evidence appears inadequate to support a recommendation for daily intake of dairy foods to promote bone health in the general population of the United States."[32] Having strong bones is about much more than just calcium. We require vigorous exercise, adequate vitamin D, and a diet rich in many micronutrients.

Heart disease and dementia are consequences of aging.

FALSE

Interestingly, heart disease as a major cause of disability and death is a recent phenomenon in human history. Heart disease has identifiable causes, and populations whose lifestyle practices do not create these causes do not have heart disease. Cultures around the world eating a vegetable-rich diet have no recorded heart disease, including hundreds of thousands of rural Chinese.[33] In addition to heart disease, diets that are high in animal fats and low in vitamins, minerals, fruits, and green vegetables also have been shown to be related to the incidence of dementia.[34]

What criteria do you use for accepting new knowledge? Much of the information that I am presenting to you may be difficult to accept because it questions conventional wisdom and accepts only what can be proven with scientific evidence. Our cognitive models are based on our perceptions and feelings, not on actual facts. It is not the situation itself that determines what we feel, but rather it is the way we think about the situation. Learning this material might require you to change your way of thinking and, therefore, change your subconscious cognitive model. It will happen gradually and naturally as you go through the exercises and as your health improves as a result of your new eating patterns.

In the realm of health education and health care, misinformation abounds. Misinformation actually works hand in hand with self-deception. Countless diets advertise that you can eat all of the foods you love and still lose weight. Consequently, why would anyone want to completely revamp his or her diet? It seems like it would be far easier to eat less of something that you love than it would be to switch to eating something that you may not currently like. The problem is that, in practice, this has been proven not to work.

Studies have shown that portion control diets result in significant weight loss that is maintained over five years for fewer than three people out of 100.[35] These diets are doomed to fail because they do not satisfy our biological need for nutrients, and we continue to crave more calories than we actually require. In addition, these diets reinforce the low-nutrient eating that we now know causes most medical problems in modern countries. They are founded on weak science and perpetuate nutritional myths. To become healthy, disease-proof, and permanently thin, you can't escape the necessity of eating large amounts of nutrient-rich, healthful food.

Why we believe things that we know are not true

If we were completely rational, all of our decisions would be based squarely on either facts or evidence. But, as we know, we often are not rational, and even people with a complete command of the facts will not make sound decisions. Consider addicted smokers. They can tell you all of the reasons why smoking is harmful, yet, for reasons they cannot articulate, they simultaneously believe they are better off continuing their addiction. Both their emotional and physical addictions prejudice their judgment, and they make rationalizations to believe something that clearly is not true.

Before we judge them, it should be noted that most Americans have heard over and over again that fruits and vegetables are the most healthful foods and that we need to eat larger amounts of them to protect against heart disease and cancer. Nevertheless, people typically dismiss or diminish the importance of this message. Their subconscious is not comfortable with change, and their subconscious wins. Inertia, the resistance of our ego to a change in its state of prior beliefs, prevails.

All of our actions and decisions are governed by our core beliefs. Our core beliefs define the limits of what we will and will not do. You may need to change your core beliefs in order to get healthy. At this point, you know that eating more vegetables has health benefits, but you may not really feel that this lifesaving information will give you control of your health destiny, save you from suffering with pain, and add many quality years to your life. Your subconscious mind hasn't accepted it yet. For many people, the partial knowledge that they have acquired is in conflict with their core beliefs. They are unable to accept it, so their awareness of it dims and, with it, the ability to make the changes.

Our self-deceptions often lead us into absurd situations that are completely obvious to outside observers. Many people blame the media and big business for the current state of the American diet. The truth, however, is that Americans are self-deceived. There is nothing that prohibits us from choosing healthful foods, but contradictions often arise between the subconscious and rational portions of our minds. We are prone to believe what we want to, regardless of the evidence. Our brains are masters at suppressing facts.

Changing our ingrained habits requires that we operate for a period of time with cognitive dissonance. Cognitive dissonance is a psychological term describing the uncomfortable tension that may result from having conflicting thoughts, or from engaging in behavior that conflicts with one's beliefs. It usually results in the filtering of new information that conflicts with what one already believes. When it comes to choosing new eating habits and developing new taste preferences, cognitive dissonance needs to be recognized so we can get over it and progress. We must face the facts, accept our discomfort, and work through it.

Your subconscious might not be comfortable with the changes you are trying to make, but you have to hang in there until the change feels natural. Your taste preferences will change with time. The first step, of course, is getting started. In recognizing your discomfort, you will be able to acknowledge it and move on, so that you move one step closer to taking control of your health.

DEVELOPING A TASTE FOR HEALTH

....

Long established beliefs about health and food have created a cognitive model for our society, and that model affects your eating habits. One of the key principles you need to learn that goes counter to this cognitive model is taste subjectivity. Your tastes can be changed. We live in a food-obsessed society. Most people believe that their sense of taste represents something that is particularly unique to them. This is not the case; in recent years, our taste preferences have been hijacked and altered by manufacturers of artificial foods.

Consider the following statement: "Healthy foods don't taste good."

Is that true? Inherently, no, but many people in our society would agree. If taste was something fixed and unchangeable, then this would create quite a problem for those who want to eat healthfully. Being healthy would require us to eat things that do not taste good. Being healthy, therefore, would be an unnatural and illogical state. However, taste is not fixed. It is a learned response. The idea that a food "can grow on you" is true.

Our tastes are the result of our bodies adapting to the foods that we eat on a regular basis. Before the advent of refrigeration and global commerce, we only could eat foods that were grown locally. Notice how people in different regions have different tastes. Are they born with different taste preferences than we are? No, their tastes have simply adapted to the foods in their region.

What does the phrase "healthy foods don't taste good" really mean? By itself, the phrase means that people have adapted their taste preferences to prefer the unhealthful foods they generally eat. However, what if they could change their preferences so that they would not only enjoy, but also prefer, the taste of healthful foods? This can happen as you put this program to the test. In the beginning, as you force yourself to eat these healthful foods, you will begin to enjoy them more. As you complete the "Exercises with Food," sample new recipes, and slowly decrease your intake of processed and other unhealthful foods, you will notice that your taste preferences will change. It's one of the many amazing changes that you will see by making the high-nutrient diet an integral part of your lifestyle.

> *"We can't solve problems by using the same kind of thinking we used when we created them."*
>
> —Albert Einstein

These words of wisdom from Einstein can be applied to your eating habits. The thought process that caused you to gain excess weight will not be helpful as you try to lose it. You must be willing to let go of the old ideas that no longer serve you and never really did. Your health and weight are governed by the law of cause and effect.

Most people don't fail because of a lack of effort. The most common mistake that prevents people from achieving their goals is that they do the same thing over and over, illogically expecting a different result. They get locked into a single way of looking at things. Taking a different approach requires us to think differently. Here, it requires us to rethink what we consider a new way of eating. For a moment, consider the old definition of the standard grain-based diet and the tenets of my nutrient-dense, vegetable-based style of eating:

HIGH-NUTRIENT DIET	STANDARD DIET
Vegetable-based	Grain-based
Lots of beans, nuts, and seeds	Lots of dairy and meats
At least four fresh fruits daily	Lots of refined sweeteners
Oils used sparingly	Oils used liberally
Animal products minimized (zero to two times per week)	Animal products emphasized (two to three times per day)
Focused on nutrient-dense calories	Focused on nutrient-poor calories

You can see that a major overhaul is required in your way of thinking to strive for a healthful diet. However, with time and focus, eating the high-nutrient way will become what tastes good to you.

Inflexible palate syndrome

The notion that food preferences can't be changed is so common that I have given it a name: inflexible palate syndrome. An inflexible palate is one that does not tolerate new foods. It prevents people from even starting to change their lives. They believe that they can't eat better because they don't like the taste of healthful food. But remember, our tastes are subjective, learned responses to the foods that we eat on a regular basis. By systematically changing the foods that we eat, we can reprogram our perceived taste responses. By following the guidelines in this book, this syndrome can be eradicated. The menus and recipes presented in *3 Steps to Incredible Health, Volume 2* can be a tremendous help in this regard.

Inflexible palate syndrome is an impediment. An impediment blocks you from achieving a desired goal. There may be many impediments on your road to better health. Good health, however, is governed by the law of cause and effect. When you start eating healthful whole foods, the desired effect will follow. The underlying habits required to achieve good health are all learnable skills.

Reprogramming yourself

As a society, we have programmed ourselves to eat in a way that is unnatural and harmful. We mistakenly prefer the tastes of harmful foods. The most natural and healthful way of eating now seems strange and eludes us. The benefits of eating natural foods, as opposed to processed foods, seem obvious, yet they are lost to many. Here are a few of the common excuses that I hear from people:

- "It takes too much effort and time to prepare fresh food."

- "I don't like the taste of fruits and vegetables."

- "People will think I am strange if I eat this way."

Even if you don't voice these objections, you may still be thinking them. They may form the core of your inner dialogue. This kind of talk is not useful. Its purpose is to prevent you from taking action. It is a type of learned helplessness; you don't believe you can succeed, so you create a rationale for not trying. Right now, resolve to fight these thoughts when they enter your head. These excuses are not based on facts. They are opinions formed before adequate knowledge was available, and as you now know, knowledge is the cornerstone to success. Your internal programming and fixed beliefs can make you fail before you even start. This internal programming operates outside of your conscious awareness, yet it influences your thoughts and actions.

Psychologists tell us that both preconceived notions and the inner dialogue that resists change to a preexisting belief are automatic thoughts. An automatic thought is an unconscious process that determines how we interpret the events of our lives. In many people, these thoughts are negative, pessimistic, and completely illogical. They persist because they operate beyond awareness and because they go completely unquestioned and unchallenged. Our automatic thoughts are the result of our core beliefs, and our core beliefs establish our perceived boundaries of what we can and cannot do.

The key to reprogramming yourself is to select an activity that elicits the desired objective, and then perform this activity habitually. As you continue to perform this activity, your skill will improve, your brain will reprogram to the preferred wiring, and your desired outcome will manifest itself. Your brain is not only flexible and adaptable, but it also will restructure itself to accommodate whatever lifestyle you wish to create.

For years, athletes have done visualization exercises to rehearse their physical specialties completely in their minds. They use their minds to train their bodies. Scientists have discovered how this works. In one study, subjects were instructed to raise their arms while their brains were scanned. They were then instructed to simply think about the act. The limbic brain patterns were identical. The athlete simply learns how to reproduce the same limbic pattern while she is performing it. Similarly, using PET (Photo-Emission Tomography) scan technology, neuroscientists have observed that people with similar lifestyles and circumstances have similarly structured brains.

Consider taxicab drivers in London. London streets are very complex. Taxi drivers go through extensive training and are required to know the best route and alternates between any two addresses. When the brains of these taxi drivers were scanned, researchers discovered that they all had unusually large hippocampus regions. The hippocampus is the part of the brain used to handle spatial orientation and navigation. What was even more interesting was that the size of the hippocampus was proportional to the time that the individual had driven the cab. The activity or skill of being able to drive a cab through a complex maze like London caused the hippocampus to continuously grow, long after the period of active study ended.[36] For both athletes and these taxi drivers, practicing their skills changed their brains. For you, practicing how you want to eat will change how your brain works in relation to your food preferences.

Just as you cannot expect to develop a perfect tennis swing or learn how to play a musical instrument without both good instruction and a tremendous amount of practice, you cannot hope to transform your health without the ongoing process of putting your new knowledge into action. Moving in the right direction, improving the way you eat, and learning how to handle social situations that encourage bad habits are all part of an ongoing process of healthy change. It is a process that requires time and effort and the ability to learn from mistakes. As the saying goes, practice makes perfect. It is not enough simply to know what to do. You need to do it. You need to practice preparing recipes and eating super-healthful meals until you reach the point where they satisfy your desire for pleasurable eating.

Anyone who has become accomplished at demanding activities, such as sports and music, will tell you that it can be difficult to learn new things. It is not easy to develop new habits, and there is no such thing as a shortcut to developing new skills and expertise. Likewise, it takes practice and perseverance to eat healthfully.

When you do something over and over, it creates a pathway in the brain that makes it easier and more comfortable to repeat it again later. That is one reason why it is so hard to change a person with ingrained bad habits. For example, I would rather teach someone who never played tennis before how to properly swing a racket than to try to teach someone who has been playing for years and swings incorrectly. That's why teaching this high-nutrient eating to children from an early age is such a good idea. They don't have the bad habits ingrained, so it is easier for them to accept. However, while change may be difficult, it is not impossible. What is needed is a strong desire and motivation to change, a willingness to be uncomfortable, and a determination to work on it until you get it right.

The more you make healthful meals, and the more days you link together eating healthful foods, the more your brain will naturally prefer to eat this way. Your taste for healthful foods will develop. It has been shown that a new food needs to be eaten about fifteen times for it to become a preferred food. The more days you eat healthfully, the more you will lose your addiction to unhealthful, stimulating substances. With time, you will look forward to—and prefer eating— a diet that is more natural and wholesome.

Your diet, your choice

One day, I asked myself why I eat the way I do. What is my motivation? What do I get out of it? So what if I die younger. Why not just enjoy all the processed food our high-tech, modern world has to offer? Why not eat cheeseburgers, fries, soda, and ice cream for lunch, and take my chances with an earlier death? At least I will enjoy the time I am alive, right?

In thinking about it, I realized that I actually enjoy eating the way I do. I believe I get more pleasure from eating than people who live on unhealthful food because I've learned to appreciate the tastes and flavors of natural foods, and I know I'm doing something good for myself. I would eat this way anyway, even if there was a slight decrease in the pleasure of eating, but after years of eating like this, I prefer it. The fact that it is good for me is certainly the largest attraction, but health-destroying foods are not appealing to me anymore. However, I have complete freedom to eat anything I want, and if I occasionally want to eat something unhealthful, I do. But, over the years, I have found that I desire unhealthful foods less and less because I do not feel well after eating them. Plus, the taste is never as pleasurable as I anticipate it will be.

I and others have developed great tasting, healthful alternatives to tempting but unhealthful foods. These alternatives make it easier to choose to eat right. I do not feel deprived. I eat the way I am advocating that you eat. I am not overweight, and I am not on a diet. I may not eat perfectly all the time, but I have balanced pleasure and health in my diet so that I am not sacrificing one to have the other. I eat this way for a lot of reasons:

- I enjoy this way of eating. It tastes great, and I like to eat lots of food.

- I want control of my health, and I want complete assurance that I will not suddenly have a heart attack or stroke.

- I enjoy living too much. I love sports, travel, entertainment, exercise, my work, and my family, and I want to maintain my youthful vigor and enjoyment of life.

- I feel well eating this way and do not like the way I feel, the way I sleep, my digestion, or my mental energy when I do not eat this way.

- I want to live longer and without medical interference, pain, and unnecessary suffering in my later years.

Eating healthfully is an option, a choice. You have the right to care for yourself as you choose. Others may choose to engage in risky behaviors, using the rationale that a pleasure-seeking, life-shortening option is preferable. The fallacy is that people who smoke, drink, take drugs, or eat dangerous foods think that they are enjoying life more. In fact, they enjoy it less because the harmful results of their addictive behaviors remain long after the temporary pleasure has vanished.

Toxic habits and disease-causing foods actually inhibit your ability to get pleasure from eating. A healthier body means stronger taste buds. Your taste buds become less sensitive from chronic excess exposure to sweets, salt, and other unhealthful substances. Food then tastes bland. You lose the ability to appreciate the subtle variety of flavors in natural foods, and you become dependent on using excess sugar and salt.

Eat healthfully, and over time you will prefer eating healthfully. Delicious, even gourmet recipes can be designed for a high-nutrient diet. It is almost insane to commit suicide with a disease-causing diet.

People who have adopted my high-nutrient advice have reversed longstanding conditions, including autoimmune diseases, diabetes, headaches, and heart disease, and have been brought back from the brink of death. All this simply by changing the way they eat. This experience of seeing the results of thousands of people transform their lives suggests that you have an opportunity to age more slowly and add healthy years to your life. Sadly, a very large number of people are simply unable to even attempt this change. Their habits now control them, and they are no longer in total control of their lives. I urge you—don't be one of them.

EXERCISES WITH FOOD: THE WORKOUT

Now that you have warmed up to healthful, high-nutrient, whole foods, it is time to turn the workout routine up a notch. I want you to start eating so many more vegetables and fruits that they become the foundation of your diet.

In this workout, we will focus on palate stretching exercises. Instead of stretching your biceps with barbells, you will be stretching your palate and digestive system with a variety of raw and conservatively cooked, natural foods.

It's okay if you don't love the taste of these foods at first. When you eat a meal, you expect to like what you are eating. However, when you are exercising, it is okay not to like the exercise while you are doing it because you are not exercising for its own sake. You are looking forward to the increase in muscle or endurance that comes afterwards. When trying a new healthful but unfamiliar dish, you might not enjoy the taste at first. You might even think that you will never enjoy it. More likely, you just need to give your taste buds a little time to get used to it.

We can call this exercise "eating without taste expectations." Going through this phase is a necessary step for people who want to create great health. It is helpful while doing the palate stretching to concentrate on the physical benefits of the foods that you are eating. Habitually stretching your palate will increase your exposure to healthful foods until over time, you will prefer their tastes.

EXERCISE 3

Take the half-pound of vegetables and half-pound of fruit that you are eating daily and increase them to one pound each per day. The pound of vegetables can be raw or cooked. Eating two salads daily—one of vegetables and one of fruit or whatever combination you feel like— is not too much. To help you meet your vegetable goal, eat a bowl of vegetable bean soup or a vegetable bean casserole each day. The recipes in *3 Steps to Incredible Health, Volume 2* can help you along the way. Try some of the delicious salad dressing recipes with your salads, or use them as dips for raw vegetables.

EXERCISE 4

As you add more volume to your diet, also change the types of fruits and vegetables that you are eating. Alternate at least two different fruits and two different vegetables in your diet each week. Also, I encourage you as part of this exercise to try a fruit or vegetable that you rarely eat or have never tried. This is a good opportunity to see the palate stretching in action as you realize that your tastes can change. Grocery stores today have plenty of variety in their produce departments that most likely contain something you've not yet discovered. Be adventurous; stretch your palate and your experience in an effort to have a more complete diet.

Workout goals

- Eat one pound of fruit and one pound of vegetables daily. The pound of vegetables should be a combination of raw and cooked.

- Eat a bowl of vegetable bean soup or a vegetable bean casserole or stew daily. You can choose from my recipes or from low- or no-sodium varieties from the store.

- Try some of my delicious salad dressing recipes with your salads and raw vegetables.

- Alternate at least two different fruits and two different vegetables in your diet each week. Experiment with new fruits and vegetables.

Inevitable roadblocks

As we have discussed, there are many impediments on the road to becoming truly healthy. For many people, they can include having low self-esteem, lacking a support group, feeling hesitant about giving up foods, and not wanting to take the time to gain the knowledge necessary for change. Place a score of 1 to 10 on the lines below to indicate the strength of that obstacle in your life:

_____ I don't know if I can learn to like the taste of healthful foods.

_____ I don't know if I can give up unhealthful foods that I like.

_____ I don't know if my family will eat healthful food.

_____ I don't want to eat differently from other people.

_____ I don't know if my friends and relatives will like me if I eat this way.

_____ I don't know how I will eat in business, traveling, and social situations.

_____ I don't know if I can manage the time to prepare foods like this.

_____ I don't know if I can find enough time to exercise regularly.

_____ I don't know if I can make the time to shop for
food.

_____ I don't know if I can learn to cook healthful food.

_____ I don't like to cook.

_____ I can't afford to spend more money on food than I
do now.

_____ I hear so much conflicting information about
nutrition, I don't know what's true.

_____ Diets never worked for me in the past, so I would
rather not try.

_____ I can't lose weight no matter what I do.

_____ Other roadblock _____

_____ **Total Roadblock Score**

People always can come up with an excuse to avoid something that
is difficult to do. The subconscious mind is great at this, but a strong
desire and commitment on your part to achieve your health and
weight goals can silence these objections.

With planning and support, you can reduce the intensity of each of the roadblocks, and eventually eliminate them.

Revisit this page over the course of following this plan, both when you are feeling comfortable and when you are encountering difficulties. When you are hitting a rough patch, remind yourself that you are in control. You have consciously evaluated the difficulties, and, while that doesn't remove them, it should stop you from using them as a crutch. When you revisit this page during a comfortable time, score these roadblocks again. You will see the total roadblock score decrease, indicating how gaining the knowledge and living the plan is changing the way your thought process works.

THE COMPLEXITIES OF HUNGER

We commonly call the feeling of wanting or needing to eat "hunger," but to understand hunger, we need to address four important considerations: volume, nutrients, calories, and addictions. Many diets fail because they only focus on one of these—calories. The high-nutrient diet is the only dietary program that takes all four into consideration.

1. VOLUME—You must consume a sufficient amount of food, and fiber from that food, to physically feel satiated.

2. NUTRIENTS—You must consume enough nutrients in your food to enable your body to meet its biological need to thrive. Even if you have adequate volume, if it's from low-nutrient food, your body will have a nutrient deficit, and you will feel that you require more food.

3. CALORIES—You will be driven to overconsume calories unless you get enough volume and nutrients for your body to feel satiated.

4. ADDICTIONS—You must put an end to your addictions to food, which often manifest themselves in discomfort and cravings. If you don't, your body will not be able to regulate its caloric needs appropriately.

As you can see, none of these dimensions of what we call hunger functions independently. If one dimension is not tended to, the others will be thrown off. Portion-control diets attempt to limit calories without regard to nutrients or volume, hunger is never fully satisfied, and the undernourished dieter ends up giving in to the overwhelming compulsion to eat more. We have discussed the importance of nutrients and calories and how the two work together. Now, we will address the main reason that people eat too much and become overweight: food addiction.

Emotional addictions

Lots of people are overweight, and most of them know being overweight is not good for their health. Often, their friends and family and even their doctors have advised them to lose weight, but they can't. They have tried various diets and simply can't stick with them.

People often overeat for emotional comfort. It can bring fleeting pleasure. Food can be a drug-like outlet to dull the pain and dissatisfaction of life, but, like drug or alcohol use, it is never a good long-term solution. It only winds up complicating things further. What people of all body weights really want is to feel proud of themselves. This cannot be achieved by overeating and eating unhealthfully. Packing on additional pounds leads to more guilt and self-hate and, subsequently, more overeating to dull the pain. The solution to this cycle must include more than just menus and diet plans; an emotional overhaul is needed.

Your eating for comfort has to be replaced with other outlets that build self-esteem and offer solace in emotionally healthy ways. For many people, these outlets can include feeling proud of yourself for improving your health through exercise, for kindness to others, for doing a job well, for developing a new skill, and for making more choices that will improve your future health. Losing weight can be a powerful boost to your self-confidence and self-esteem. The more reasons you have to feel good about yourself, the increased likelihood you will succeed in every aspect of your life. Your new attitude must be one that lets go of the idea that you are stuck with your lot in life and that you can't change things. You can. When you are overweight and you lose weight, you can see it, as can everyone around you. It is a visible representation that you have changed and have taken back control of your life.

Once you experience how effectively the high-nutrient diet can transform your health, drop excess weight, and dramatically heighten your emotional well-being, you will stop coming up with rationalizations why the effort is not worth it. However, to realize those rewards, you first must put this program into action. Getting healthy takes considerable focus and effort. You need to plan and put time into this. Of course, it is easier to eat processed and convenient foods and claim you are too busy to squeeze exercise into your schedule, but the effort to do what it takes is well worth it. It will allow you to transform your health and set you free to enjoy a much more pleasurable life. When you make the commitment to take proper care of yourself and put out the effort, you take back control.

Emotional issues are tied into the act of eating for many people, so there is no need to feel alone in experiencing them. It is helpful to have a friend or a social support network so you can share and discuss these topics.

Food addiction and the fat cycle

Almost every person eating the standard, toxic, American diet develops strong physical addictions. It is crucial to address and resolve these addictions. When a heavy coffee drinker stops drinking coffee, he feels ill, experiencing headaches and weakness, and even feels nervous and shaky. Fortunately, these symptoms resolve slowly over four to six days. Discomfort after stopping an addictive substance is called withdrawal, and it is significant because it represents detoxification, or a biochemical healing that is accomplished after the substance is withdrawn. It is nearly impossible to cleanse the body of a harmful substance without experiencing the discomfort of withdrawal. Humans have a tendency to want to avoid discomfort. They continue their toxic habits to avoid unpleasant withdrawal symptoms. When we discontinue consuming healthful substances, such as broccoli or spinach, we do not experience discomfort. We feel nothing. Only unhealthful, toxic substances are addicting, and, therefore, these are the only substances that cause discomfort when you stop consuming them. Their addictive potential is proportional to their toxicity.

Uncomfortable sensations are often the signal that repair is under way and the removal of toxins is occurring. Although it may be difficult to adjust to this way of thinking, feeling ill temporarily can be seen as a sign that you are getting well. That cup of coffee may make you feel better temporarily, but any stimulating substance that makes you feel better quickly, or gives you immediate energy, is hurtful, not healthful. Any substance that has that immediate effect is toxic and called a stimulant. Healthful foods do not induce stimulation. When you meet your needs for nutrients and sleep, your body will naturally feel well and fully energized, without the need for stimulation.

The more you search for fast, temporary relief with a candy bar, a can of soda, or a bag of chips, the more you inhibit the healing, detoxification process. Your body becomes increasingly toxic as you give it more low-nutrient calories. Calories consumed without the accompanying nutrients that aid in their assimilation and metabolism lead to a buildup of toxic substances in the cells that promote cellular aging and disease. Eating low-nutrient calories increases dangerous free-radical activity within the cells and allows for the build-up of cellular waste. These low-nutrient calories also increase other toxic materials in the body, such as advanced glycation end products (AGEs). AGEs affect nearly every type of cell and molecule in the body, and are major factors in aging and age-related chronic diseases. Their production is markedly accelerated in diabetics, and they are believed to play a causative role in the neurologic and vascular complications of the disease.

AGEs are the result of a chain of chemical reactions and may be formed externally to the body by overcooking foods or inside the body though cellular metabolism. They form at a slow rate in the normal body and may accumulate with time, but their formation can be accelerated by your eating habits. The secret to aging more slowly and remaining youthful is to prevent the accumulation of AGEs in the body.

Dry cooking methods such as baking, roasting, and broiling cause sugars to combine with proteins to form AGEs, while water-based cooking, such as steaming and boiling, does not. AGEs are highest in burnt and browned foods, and are highest in overcooked animal products, but these compounds also can build up in cells from the consumption of low-nutrient calories, especially calories from sweets. So, eating both overcooked foods and low-nutrient foods leads to the buildup of AGEs and ages us faster. When you eat a diet that is based on toxic and addictive foods—such as salt, fried foods, snack foods, processed and barbequed meats, and sugary drinks, you not only build up free radicals and AGEs in your cells, you also set the stage for feeling ill when you are not digesting food. Unhealthful food allows your body to create waste byproducts that must be removed by the liver and other organs. Only when digestion ends can the body fully take advantage of the opportunity to remove toxins. While the body is digesting, it can't go through this detoxification process effectively.

When detoxification begins, people often feel queasiness or malaise. Eating something restarts digestion and shuts down the detoxification process, making the bad feelings go away. The lower the nutritional quality of your diet, the worse you will feel if you try to stop eating food for a few hours. You will only feel normal while your digestive tract is busy.

Toxic hunger

After years of eating a poor diet, detoxifying your body can be both physically and psychologically difficult. The latter is involved because people often think that, since eating makes them feel better, the symptoms of detoxification are actually hunger. This leads to one continuous eating binge all day. It is no wonder that 80 percent of Americans are overweight. Every few hours, they are compelled to put something in their mouths. They may feel better temporarily from that chocolate-chip cookie or pretzel, but they never really get rid of their uncomfortable symptoms. The symptoms come back again and again.

I call these detoxification (withdrawal) symptoms toxic hunger. It will recur whenever digestion ceases, not when an individual is truly hungry and has a biological need for calories. Toxic hunger keeps coming back to haunt you every time your digestive apparatus is no longer busy digesting. Eating a large meal with lots of excess calories can keep the digestive tract busy for hours and hours, keeping these symptoms at bay until it is time for the next meal. Because you feel the desire to eat so frequently, you will become overweight, and, in the process, your opportunity for a long life and disease-free future is lost.

Food addiction affects almost all Americans. It takes superior nutrition to lose the symptoms of toxic hunger. Toxic hunger makes it almost impossible to reduce portion sizes, cut back on calories, count points, or follow other typical dieting strategies. You can't easily stop overeating when you are a food addict. A person can't be expected to eat less food when they feel so bad when they do. Unless people are informed, they mistake the withdrawal symptoms they feel for hunger, or claim they have hypoglycemia and they simply can't help eating too frequently and too much. Once you address your addictions and use this knowledge to help yourself through the detoxification process, you will be able to more easily, efficiently, and pleasurably address your nutrient and caloric requirements.

Toxic hunger is a physical addiction to an unhealthful, low-micro-nutrient diet. Its symptoms are generally feelings that we have been taught to interpret as hunger. However, they are actually signs of your body's toxicity.

SYMPTOMS OF TOXIC HUNGER

- headaches
- weakness, shakiness and fatigue
- stomach cramping
- lightheadedness

- esophageal spasms
- growling stomach
- irritability and inability to concentrate

These uncomfortable symptoms are experienced to different degrees by different individuals. Sugary foods with a high glycemic index can fuel these symptoms and the toxic hunger eating frenzy, but consuming too many animal products can do it, too. Americans are now accustomed to eating animal products, including beef, chicken, eggs, and cheese, at every meal, but eating such a high quantity of these very-high-protein foods can overload the liver's ability to eliminate excessive nitrogenous wastes. The excessive consumption of animal proteins and the elevated amount of waste products puts a stress on your body's detoxification channels, and you wind up not feeling well—or detoxifying more—between meals.

Some people are more sensitive to this excess nitrogen than others. It is not unusual to find people who feel forced to eat a diet rich in protein and animal products. Otherwise, they feel too ill. They must remain on a continual high-protein binge all day. They feel terrible if they try to stop eating high-protein foods or if they delay eating. These individuals may feel better when eating animal products at regularly spaced intervals, but this is the same as drinking more coffee to feel better. It leads to more and more addictive symptoms, and they never get better. Just like the caffeine addict, they may have to feel worse for a short time for these symptoms to resolve. Even though the overeating of animal protein causes the problem, the high-protein food also temporarily allows them to feel better and to feel better longer after the meal because high-protein foods take longer to digest and can delay the discomfort of withdrawal.

Eating again to remove those uncomfortable feelings never gets you off the overeating merry-go-round. You can have another cup of coffee or slice of cheese in an attempt to feel better, but it is this cycle that caused you to become overweight and suffer these ill feelings in the first place. To get rid of the toxic hunger symptoms that drive overeating behavior, you may have to feel uncomfortable for a few days to resolve the issue. I often have people make a gradual change in their diet to minimize the discomfort, but eventually as they are able to change the diet more and more, they lose the hypoglycemic symptoms and are able to feel comfortable delaying eating or eating less. This is a necessary first step for them to get back in control of their overeating. Toxic hunger is the main reason people fail on diets. Toxic hunger is a primary cause of obesity and overweight problems in the modern world. We have adopted a toxic diet, and because of it, we are forced to overeat.

True hunger and health

The high-nutrient diet can set you free from your food addictions and allow you to lose your toxic hunger. The food cravings will end, and you will be able to stop overeating. You will be back in contact with true hunger. When you achieve that, you will be able to accurately sense the calories you need to maintain your health and lean body.

I want to reiterate that as you adopt the high-nutrient diet, it is common to go through an adjustment period in which you experience fatigue, weakness, lightheadedness, headaches, gas, and other mild symptoms. This generally lasts less than a week. Don't panic or buy into the myth that to get relief you need more heavy or stimulating foods, such as high-protein foods, sweets, or coffee.

The feelings associated with these symptoms are not how true hunger feels. It is our unhealthy tendency to eat without experiencing true hunger that has caused us to become overweight in the first place. To become overweight, a person's food cravings, recreational eating, and other addictive drives have come into play. Poor nutrition causes these cravings, and superior nutrition helps normalize or remove them. You will no longer feel the need to overeat when you eat healthfully.

True hunger is not felt in the stomach or the head. These symptoms melt away with time. When you eat healthfully and don't overeat, you eventually are able to sense true hunger and accurately assess your caloric needs. Once your body attains a certain level of better health, you will begin to feel the difference between true hunger and just eating due to desire, boredom, stress, or withdrawal symptoms. The best way to understand true hunger is to experience it for yourself. It has three primary characteristics:

- a sensation in your throat
- increased salivation
- a dramatically heightened taste sensation

Being in touch with true hunger will help you reach your ideal weight, and you also will feel well whether you eat, delay eating, or skip a meal. Almost all of my patients who suffered with headaches and so-called "hypoglycemia" have gotten well permanently following my nutritional recommendations.

How true hunger works

People generally snack between meals to satisfy toxic hunger and food cravings, or they consume empty calories and toxic food while eating for recreational purposes. Recreational eating is eating because you are in a social setting or simply because there is food around you. Recreational eating still can occur without satisfying toxic hunger or true hunger. Sometimes people—including me—just enjoy eating good-tasting food when it is offered, even though we are not feeling any symptoms directing us to eat. When most people eat in this way, they do it with junk food, not healthful, natural foods. The way we can reduce recreational eating is by experiencing how much more enjoyable it is to eat when we are really hungry. Then we find that the food tastes much better. This heightened taste sensation that accompanies true hunger gives us terrific feedback to inhibit overeating behavior so we can actually get more pleasure out of our diet. Delaying eating, to the point when true hunger is experienced, makes even ordinary foods taste great and extraordinary foods taste even better.

In our present toxic food environment, we have lost the ability to connect with the body signals that tell us how much food we actually need. We have become slaves to withdrawal symptoms and eat all day long when there is no biological need for calories. This is not in harmony with our natural physiology. In an environment of healthful food choices, we do not feel any signals to eat until hormonal and neurological messengers indicate that glycogen reserves in the liver are decreased and lean body mass will soon be used as an energy source. Our bodies have the beautifully orchestrated ability to tell us exactly how much to eat to maintain an ideal weight for our long-term health. These signals are what I call true hunger. This name also differentiates it from toxic hunger, which is what everyone else refers to simply as hunger. Even some medical textbooks make this mistake. Most Americans have not felt true hunger since they were toddlers.

Feeding yourself to satisfy true hunger cannot cause weight gain. If you only ate when truly hungry, it would be almost impossible to become overweight. True hunger is a signal to eat to maintain your muscle mass. Eating to satisfy true hunger does not put fat on your body. Excessive fat stores are developed only from eating outside of your body's true hunger demands. When you get back in touch with true hunger, you instinctively will know how much to eat. When you exercise more, you will get more and more frequent hunger; when you exercise less, you will get much less hunger. Your body will become a precise calorie-measuring computer and steer you in the right direction, just from eating the amount that feels right and makes food taste best.

True hunger is not uncomfortable. It does not involve your stomach fluttering or cramping. When you feel it, you know it is a normal reaction that signals a need for food. It signals that the body is physiologically ready to digest, and the digestive glands have regained their capacity to secrete enzymes appropriately. It makes food taste much better when you eat, and it makes eating much more pleasurable. People are consistently amazed at how good the simplest foods can taste when they are truly hungry.

I have observed this changing perception of hunger in thousands of individuals who adopted my high-nutrient diet. I have documented this discovery in scientific studies and explained the biochemistry behind it. It is the pillar supporting and strengthening my teachings that removes the addictive prison of overeating.

True hunger requires no special food to satisfy it. It is satisfied by eating almost anything. You can't crave some particular food and call it hunger. A craving, by definition, is an addictive drive, not something felt by a person who is not an addict. Remember, almost all Americans are addicted to their toxic habits. A disease-causing diet is addicting. A health-supporting diet is not.

To consume the exact number of calories necessary to maintain a lean body mass that will prolong life, you must get rid of toxic hunger and get back in touch with true hunger. If you eat when hungry and don't eat when not hungry, you will never have to diet or be overweight again. You do not have to carry around a calculator and a scale to figure out how much to eat. A healthy body will give you the correct signals. You only will desire the amount of calories you actually require.

Getting enough volume

Our hunger drive craves volume. A key skill that you are developing is the ability to eat large volumes of raw and cooked high-nutrient, low-calorie foods every single day. This means eating lots of vegetables. It may be helpful to look again at the illustration of stomachs in Chapter 5. Each is filled with the same amount of calories, but one contains those calories in the form of oil, one in the form of chicken, and one in the form of vegetables. The stomachs with the oil and chicken have a great deal of room in them, room that can enable you to easily overeat on calories. That's why filling your stomach with high-nutrient foods is so important to acquiring and maintaining a healthy weight. This leads us to a counterintuitive, but crucial rule: To lose more weight, and for better health, eat more high-volume, low-calorie foods. To lose more, eat more.

When you are actively trying to lose weight, you should strive to satisfy your volume requirements first, before addressing the other components of hunger. This may feel strange at first because you may not immediately feel satisfied by the higher volume of food. This is because you are accustomed to eating large quantities of high-calorie foods that cause a dopamine rush, a rush that low-calorie foods don't deliver. However, your body will adjust, be less dependent on the dopamine surge in the brain, and will gradually become more and more satisfied with fewer calories. Give yourself time, and use the knowledge you have gained. Striving to fulfill your body's volume and nutrient requirements can help you resolve your food cravings and toxic hunger.

The trick to get you to desire fewer calories faster is to eat a lot of these high-volume, high-nutrient foods. You are already familiar with these, since many of the foods that you have been incorporating into your diet because of their nutrient values are also great tools in meeting your volume requirements. They include:

Raw vegetables
lettuce, tomatoes, peppers, celery, endive, snow pea pods, carrots, beets, cucumbers, water chestnuts, red cabbage, onion

Fresh fruits
melons, oranges, pears, grapes, apples, kiwis, berries, papaya

Cooked green vegetables
kale, collards, Swiss chard, brussels sprouts, string beans, asparagus, broccoli, Chinese cabbage, bok choy, artichokes, okra, zucchini

Cooked non-green vegetables
mushrooms, eggplant, carrots, cauliflower, sun-dried tomatoes, onions, bean sprouts, butternut squash, spaghetti squash

On holidays and other times when you know that you will be around a lot of unhealthful foods, fill up with these high-nutrient, low-calorie foods. Never go to a party or event with an empty stomach. Eat a large salad with assorted raw vegetables and a bowl of vegetable bean soup before going to the places that may tempt your desire to eat unhealthfully. Being healthy is about being in control. You must control your hunger, and the more low-calorie, high-volume foods you consume, the less high-calorie food you will be able to eat. When you increase these super-healthful foods in your diet, you will feel less temptation, and you will be in control of your food cravings and appetite.

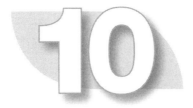

UNDERSTANDING YOUR ADDICTIONS

Most Americans are overweight. This is to be expected. People should expect to become overweight when they do not meet their needs for nutrients and volume. It turns them into food addicts, and they are forced to overeat on calories. Processed foods, low-nutrient eating, and high-protein diets based on animal products create food addictions and derail true hunger.

Understanding and managing your hunger is a critical key to creating the physical environment that will help support your efforts to earn longevity and superior health. The body's drive to feed itself is part of the design to maintain optimal health, which includes ideal weight. It is geared toward self-preservation, and its purpose is to make the body thrive. The irony is that people seem to have appetites bent on self-destruction. These are unnatural appetites.

Our ability to enjoy unhealthful foods is the result of an otherwise useful ability to adapt to a variety of environments. This was useful in the past when food was scarce. Processed and unhealthful choices were unavailable. Our tastes were designed to enable us to enjoy whatever food we could obtain from the natural environment. It helped us to distinguish foods from poisons. In today's toxic food environment, the survival drive for calories can direct us to the most calorie-concentrated processed foods. Our innate drive for calories has been shackled by the food manufacturers peddling white flour, salt, sweeteners, and artificial flavors. The more you eat low-nutrient, processed foods, the more you crave these substances. It is almost impossible not to overconsume calories and gain weight when your diet is so low in nutrients.

Dangers of salt

Salt consumption is linked to high blood pressure, blood clots, heart attacks, and stomach cancer. You might be thinking, "Wait a minute. I have low blood pressure. Why do I have to worry about salt?" The answer is that even if you have low blood pressure now, 90 percent of all Americans eventually develop high blood pressure from their high-sodium intake earlier in life. Once it is high, it is not so simple to bring it down again with the removal of salt. Instead, you wind up on medication to lower it.

Raised blood pressure is a major cause of death in the world. In most countries, 90 percent of the adult population is at risk.[37] High blood pressure is mostly the result of a poor diet, lack of exercise, and excessive salt consumption, but according to the *Journal of the American College of Cardiology*, salt consumption is a significantly bigger risk factor than the other elements.[38] If you already have high blood pressure, eating a low-salt, natural-food diet can remedy your condition and potentially save your life. Even if your blood pressure does not come down with the removal of salt, do not think salt doesn't matter for you. It may take a long time for your body to undo the damage from the many years of excessive salt intake. For those who have normal blood pressure, removing salt from your diet and following the proper dietary recommendations will mean you won't have to worry about taking medications later in life, and you will get more protection against stroke and heart attacks than medications can offer.

High sodium intake is predictive of increased death from heart attacks. A recent study of adults with pre-hypertension showed that over the ten to fifteen years that the individuals lowered their sodium intake by at least 25 percent, their risk of cardiovascular disease correspondingly fell 25 percent. The conclusion is that consuming a high amount of sodium will put you at a greater risk for heart disease and a shortened life.[39] In another recent study, high sodium intake was predictive of coronary heart disease and mortality from heart attacks, independent of other risk factors, including blood pressure. This means that it is not just about raising blood pressure. More and more direct evidence is emerging that salt is harmful to the heart in other ways.[40] Salt also causes calcium and other trace minerals to be leached from your body, which is a contributory cause of osteoporosis. As excess salt is removed via the urine, other minerals such as calcium and magnesium accompany it and are lost as well.

I understand that as you follow the high-nutrient plan, increasing your intake of fruits and vegetables and decreasing your intake of animal products and saturated fats, you may be tempted to ignore the salt factor. You may say, "I'm already making these big changes. I can't deal with taking salt away as well." However, there is another very important reason why we gradually reduce salt intake. Studies have shown that a certain type of stroke, called a hemorrhagic stroke, increases as heart attacks decrease in a population.

As the consumption of animal products and processed foods drops to lower levels in a population's diet, heart disease goes to lower and lower levels, potentially reaching less than 1 percent of the total causes of death. Eating a diet lower in animal products and higher in fruits and vegetables dramatically reduces the occurrence of the clots that cause heart disease and embolic strokes. However, hemorrhagic strokes are not caused by atherosclerosis (the buildup of fatty substances in arteries) and the resultant clots. These strokes are caused by a hemorrhage or rupture in a blood vessel wall that has been weakened by years of elevated blood pressure as a result of chronic high salt intake. The weakened wall ruptures and lets blood flow into, and damage, brain tissue.

Although whole food vegetarian and flexitarian diets that include the occasional or minimal use of animal products may markedly reduce the risk for coronary heart disease, diabetes, and many common cancers, the real Achilles heel of no-animal-fat (vegan) and low-animal-fat diets is this increased risk of hemorrhagic stroke at an older age. This is because animal products and processed foods contribute to plaque formation, called atherosclerosis. Atherosclerosis promotes blood clots that cause heart attacks and embolic strokes. However, this process may also thicken, and therefore protect, the small, fragile blood vessels in the brain from rupturing due to the stress from chronic high blood pressure. When a diet is high in fatty animal products, processed foods, and salt, the thickened blood vessel walls caused by the unhealthful, heart-attack-promoting diet actually protect against the occurrence of this more uncommon cause of strokes. In medical studies, higher cholesterol levels are associated with increased risk of embolic or non-ischemic strokes, but lower risk of hemorrhagic strokes.[41]

Admittedly, these types of strokes cause only a small percentage of deaths in modern countries, but that is because so many people die prematurely of heart disease or cancer that they don't live long enough to experience this additional detrimental effect of their high-salt diets. However, for those striving to maximize their life span, it is even more important to avoid a high-salt intake.

Decreasing salt, increasing taste

Now that you understand why salt must be dramatically lowered in your diet, you still may be questioning how you will do it without eating bland food every day. Part of the answer is that you won't be entirely eliminating sodium. To do that is impossible because all foods, especially vegetables, contain sodium, and this natural sodium adds to their flavor.

Up until now, you have probably never noticed this natural sodium. When our taste buds are overstimulated with too much added salt over a long period of time, our taste receptors can't sense lower levels of salt. Natural, unsalted foods seem to have less flavor. Food tastes flat without added salt, and you need to add more salt to almost everything. This is part of the addiction cycle; we build up tolerance for unhealthful substances. The good news is that you can retrain your taste buds to be more sensitive to salt when you decrease it in your diet.

Most people consume between 2000 and 8000 milligrams of salt each day. When you get rid of the salt habit, your food may taste bland for a few weeks, but you will find that your taste buds, which were deadened by the overuse of salt, gradually regain their sensitivity. You will discover tastes that you never knew existed in natural foods. Even a simple pear or a leaf of lettuce tastes better. Foods that you previously enjoyed will taste too salty.

When you eat a diet low in salt, eventually your sensitivity to salt and other tastes gets stronger. As you get accustomed to a diet that stimulates your salt-receptive taste buds less, you enjoy more flavors in natural foods. This stronger taste ability isn't just limited to the taste sensation of salt. You also will see the phenomenon at work when eating a simple strawberry or slice of red pepper. Amazingly, your taste buds become stronger when you are off salt and sugar. Try eating some plain romaine lettuce with no dressing on it now. Then eat some after reducing your salt intake and following my high-nutrient program for a month. You will be amazed at how much more flavor that plain, unseasoned piece of lettuce has.

The bottom line is that once you break your addiction to salt, you won't miss it at all, and you will find that food actually has more flavor, not less. High-nutrient eating strengthens your senses as it improves your health.

Limiting saturated fat

Autopsy studies on adult Americans who die in car accidents, unrelated to heart conditions, demonstrate that heart disease is present in the vast majority of American adults. Almost all people over the age of forty are found to have a significant amount of atherosclerosis in their coronary arteries.[42] The bottom line is: If you eat the standard American diet (SAD) or something close to it, you are likely to develop the same diseases—heart disease, high blood pressure, stroke, dementia, and cancer—that most Americans get. You cannot escape from the biological law of cause and effect. Our long-term health is determined by our food choices.

We get heart-healthy fats in their natural, high-antioxidant environment when we eat raw seeds and nuts. Indeed, avocado, nuts, and seeds are rich in fat. They may even contain a small amount of saturated fat, but their consumption is linked to substantial protection against heart disease. Unfortunately, in the American diet, fats come primarily from meat and dairy, which are saturated, and we compound the problem by the low level of food-derived antioxidants and phytochemicals we ingest.

Saturated fat comes from many food sources, including processed foods, meat, cheese, and other animal products. Thousands of scientific research studies demonstrate that saturated fat promotes both heart disease and cancer and powerfully raises cholesterol.[43] However, the avoidance of *all* fat is not the secret to protecting your heart. The secret is avoiding saturated fat, trans fat, and processed oils.[44] These fats do not contain the fat-binding sterols, phytonutrients, and antioxidants present in high-fat, whole plant foods. When people eat high-glycemic processed foods along with animal fats and low-nutrient oils, it leads to cardiovascular disease, depresses the immune system, and increases the risk of cancer.[45]

The table below shows the saturated fat in some common foods. Small amounts of saturated fat are not dangerous, but remember, you should be striving to eat significantly less saturated fat compared to most other Americans. You will see that it is possible for people to ingest thirty or even fifty grams of saturated fat each day without thinking too much about it. Comparatively, a healthful diet typically would contain less than five grams of saturated fat.

SATURATED FAT CONTENT OF COMMON FOODS[46] GRAMS OF SATURATED FAT

Cheddar cheese (4 oz.) 24

American processed cheese (4 oz.) 24

Ricotta cheese (1 cup) 20

Swiss cheese (4 oz.) 20

Chocolate candy, semisweet (4 oz.) 20

Cheeseburger large double patty 18

T-bone steak (6 oz.) 18

Braised lamb (6 oz.) 16

Pork shoulder (6 oz.) 14

Butter (2 Tbsp.) 14

Mozzarella, part skim (4 oz.) 12

Ricotta cheese, part skim (one cup) 12

Beef, ground, lean (6 oz.) 11

Ice cream, vanilla (1 cup) 10

Chicken fillet sandwich 9

Chicken thigh no skin (6 oz.) 5

Milk (whole), 3.3% fat (one cup) 5

Plain yogurt (1 cup) 5

Two eggs 4

Chicken breast (6 oz.) 3

Salmon (6 oz.) 3

Walnuts (2 oz. or 24 halves) 3

Milk, 2% fat (1 cup) 3

Tuna (6 oz.) 3

Turkey, white, no skin, (6 oz.) 2

Almonds 2 oz. (48 nuts) 2

Sunflower seeds (2 oz.) 2

Filet of flounder (6 oz.) 0.6

Filet of sole (6 oz.) 0.6

Fruits . . . . negligible

Vegetables . . . . negligible

Beans/legumes . . . . negligible

Unfortunately, since the low-nutrient, high-animal-product diet is so prevalent in the world today, it is hard to find a population with a high percentage of people who live to advanced ages. It is a myth that, in spite of eating a lot of cheese and meat, the French do not experience heart disease to the same extent that Americans do. Heart disease, stroke, and cancer still kill the vast majority of French adults, and the percentages in each category are almost identical to the United States and other western countries. The average life expectancy in the United States is 77.8 years, and in France it is 79 years, a negligible difference. The slight difference can be accounted for by the significantly fewer female smokers in France. Keep in mind that small differences in saturated fat intake will not change these statistics much and are not as critical a risk factor as low-vegetable consumption.

While consuming high amounts of saturated fat is clearly dangerous, it is not the only villain. Keep in mind that consuming fats that raise your cholesterol is only one of many factors that increase your risk of heart disease, strokes, and dementia. Excessive blood cholesterol is also the result of eating a low-nutrient diet that causes intravascular inflammation and, as a result, heightened cholesterol production due to insufficient fiber, which binds cholesterol in the digestive tract. Your cholesterol level goes up when you don't eat enough vegetables and beans. Saturated fat, and especially trans fat, drives cholesterol higher than simply eating cholesterol does. For example, eggs are high in cholesterol, but eating eggs will not raise your cholesterol as much as eating cheese because cheese is much higher in saturated fat.

Studies in the United States and Europe have established that the incidence of death by coronary heart disease is nearly two-and-a-half times higher for people with the highest 25 percent of blood cholesterol, compared with people with the lowest 25 percent. Yet the coronary heart disease mortality for the same cholesterol levels is only one-third as great in Japan and the Mediterranean.[47] In other words, a person in Scotland with the same blood cholesterol levels as a person in Catalonia, Spain, is eight times more likely to die of coronary heart disease. It is the higher intake of fruits and vegetables in the Mediterranean area that makes the difference.

LDL cholesterol (bad cholesterol) is the one we want to watch. It is very fragile and susceptible to oxidization, which means the fat is partially rotten due to a buildup of free radicals. This oxidization is a critical factor in the depositing of plaque on blood vessel walls.[48] Fruits, vegetables, beans, seeds, and nuts are our primary source of antioxidants. Consuming enough of these foods can reduce the negative effects of LDL oxidization. Again, the problem is not just saturated fat. It is this interaction between saturated fat and a low-nutrient environment that makes it a more powerful villain.

A recent study looked at the effects of a diet with more fruits and vegetables combined with a low saturated fat intake. It showed a 76 percent reduction in heart-disease-related deaths for those consuming more than five servings of fruits and vegetables per day and less than 12 percent of calories from saturated fat, compared to those with less vegetation and more saturated fat.[49] Even this small increase in fruit and vegetable consumption and mild reduction in saturated fats showed a dramatic decrease in heart-disease-related deaths. Can you imagine the heart protection that would be possible with ten servings of fruits and vegetables and less than 5 percent of calories from saturated fat? You simply do not have to develop, suffer from, and die of heart disease if you achieve superior nutrition.

Complicating the issue here regarding saturated fat is that animal foods, even the ones low in fat, are high in protein. High intake of animal protein raises blood levels of insulin-like growth factor one (IGF-1), which heightens one's risk of cancer and accelerates aging.[50] Foods that may be low in fat, such as egg whites and white meat chicken, still promote cancer since they so effectively raise IGF-1. The other confusing issue is that when studies evaluate people who consume less fat and more refined carbohydrates such as sweets, bread and pasta, they do not see a reduction in heart disease deaths because the negative effects of refined carbohydrates are just as bad as high saturated fat intake. Some have interpreted these findings to give them the license to eat more high-fat animal products. The fact that poorly designed low-fat diets are still atherogenic (causing the formation of plaque in the inner lining of arteries), in no way minimizes the risk of eating a diet rich in fats and animal products. We must recognize that both of those dietary factors are disease-promoting. By contrast, when your diet is predominantly unrefined plant foods, rich in greens, beans, seeds, and nuts, and you are free from the negative effects from the refined carbohydrates and low in both saturated fat and animal protein, you optimize longevity.

Worst meat options

Red meat and processed meats contain more saturated fat and trans fat than other animal products and are poor food choices. However, the fat issue does not tell the whole story. Scientific studies have documented that red meat has a much more pronounced association with colon cancer and pancreatic cancer compared with other animal products.[51] The consumption of red meat and processed meats on a regular basis more than doubles the risk of some cancers. Even ingesting a small amount of red meat, such as two to three ounces per day, has been shown to significantly increase the risk of cancer.[52]

Toxic nitrogenous compounds (called N-nitroso) occur in larger concentrations in red meat and processed meats. Red meat also has high haem (also spelled heme) content. Haem is an iron-carrying protein, and it has been shown to have destructive effects on the cells lining the digestive tract.[53] Processed meat, luncheon meat, barbequed meat, and red meat must not be a regular part of your diet if you are looking to maintain excellent health into your later years of life.

Eating too many animal products and not enough vegetables increases one's risk of cancer. To achieve optimal health, humans require a high exposure to the full complement of phytochemicals found in unprocessed plant matter. Eating more animal products results in a smaller percentage of calories consumed from high phytochemical vegetation such as seeds, berries, vegetables, and beans. Also, since animal products do not contain any fiber, they remain in the digestive tract longer, slowing digestive transit time and allowing heightened exposure to toxic compounds. You should reduce your consumption of animal products gradually until you're only consuming them two to three times per week. Of course, I recommend totally avoiding processed meat and barbequed meat.

Fish no health food

Many people believe they are improving their diets by eating less meat and more fish. Since fish is generally low in fat and high in beneficial omega-3 fats, many consider it an important part of a healthful diet. Studies have demonstrated that when people eat less red meat and more fish, health outcomes are improved. However, a review of the literature on fish consumption shows that eating fish is a double-edged sword because it may contain mercury and other pollutants.

In spite of the presence of valuable omega-3 fats, called EPA and DHA, nearly all fish and shellfish contain mercury and other pollutants, such as PCBs. Pollutants and mercury accumulate in fish as the polluted water is filtered through their gills. Larger fish that have lived longer have the highest levels of mercury because they've had more time to accumulate it. They may also accumulate it from all the smaller fish they have eaten, similar to the way we accumulate mercury in our tissues from the fish we eat.

If you eat fish regularly, your body is undoubtedly high in mercury. You cannot remove the mercury in fish by trimming the fat or by cooking because it is deposited throughout the fish's tissues. Mercury levels tested in patients correlate exceptionally well with the amount of fish the individuals consumed. Individuals eating fish a few times a week had blood mercury levels exceeding 5.0 micrograms, the maximum level recommended by the National Academy of Sciences. Women eating seafood more than twice per week had seven times the blood mercury levels of non-fish eaters, and children eating fish regularly had mercury levels forty times higher than the national mean.[54] Mercury can be removed from the body naturally, but it may take years for the levels to drop significantly.

The bottom line on fish is that we can no longer consider it a healthful food. Either avoid it or eat it no more than once weekly. If you do have fish, choose from types that have the lowest amounts of mercury, such as salmon, flounder, scallops, trout, or sole. Avoid swordfish, mackerel, tilefish, and shark.[55] They contain the highest mercury levels. Be aware of the location where it was caught and what type of fish it is. Never accept recreational fish from questionable waters, and never eat high-mercury content fish. It is not worth the risk.

If the consumption of toxins contained in fish has potential health risks, wouldn't it be better to get our omega-3 fats from a cleaner source? Yes. It is safer to rely on a clean, low-dose, DHA supplement, such as my DHA Purity (www.DrFuhrman.com), or a clean fish-oil supplement taken a few times a week instead of eating potentially dirty fish. Since my DHA Purity supplement is not fish-derived, you are assured of achieving adequate DHA levels without mercury and other pollutants. When buying omega-3 supplements, keep in mind that they should be purchased from a well-documented, reliably clean source, close to the date of manufacturing, and be refrigerated upon receipt.

Detriments of dairy

The consumption of cheese has skyrocketed in recent history. Dairy is the food category that contributes the most saturated fat to the American diet, and cheese and butter are now the major contributors. As you can see from the saturated fat chart, compared with the same sized piece of fowl or fish, cheese could have ten times as much saturated fat. However, the high saturated fat content of dairy is not the primary reason to limit its consumption.

Cow's milk is the perfect food for a rapidly growing calf. There is a clear association between high-growth-promoting foods such as dairy products and cancer. There is ample evidence implicating dairy consumption as a causative factor in both prostate and ovarian cancer.[56] Dairy protein boosts the amount of insulin-like growth factor (IGF-1) in the blood. IGF-1 is found in cow's milk and has been shown to occur in increased levels in the blood of individuals consuming dairy products on a regular basis. IGF-1 is known to stimulate the growth of both normal and cancer cells. Case control studies in diverse populations have shown a strong and consistent association between serum IGF-1 concentrations and prostate cancer risk.[57]

The link between lactose (milk sugar) and ovarian cancer was investigated as part of the Nurses' Health Study, which enrolled over 80,000 women. Researchers reported that women who consumed the highest amount of lactose (one or more servings of dairy per day) had a 44 percent greater risk for all types of invasive ovarian cancer than those who ate the lowest amount (three or fewer servings monthly). Skim and low-fat milk were the largest contributors to lactose consumption.[58]

Given this clear link between increased consumption of even low-fat dairy and skim milk and cancer, it is wise to reconsider dairy as an important source of calcium in the diet. This is another reason why animal source foods should be limited. When you eat sufficiently from whole plant foods, you get plenty of calcium.

High-nutrient diet vs. vegetarian diet

As you know by now, the foundation of the high-nutrient diet is the dramatically increased consumption of micronutrient-rich vegetables, fruits, beans, seeds, and nuts. Vegans (vegetarians who consume no animal products) and vegetarians (who consume dairy products and/or other animal products) can take advantage of the high-nutrient diet as long as they follow all of the protocols. Typical vegetarian and vegan diets do not include such a large amount of high-nutrient, whole plant foods, and therefore do not offer as much in terms of improved health or longevity. Vegans and vegetarians who consume a largely plant-based diet will get some of the advantages of the high-nutrient diet, but the benefits do not come primarily from the abstinence from animal products. The benefits come from eating more vegetables, beans, fruit, nuts, and seeds compared with those eating more conventionally.

Vegans and vegetarians whose diets center around processed cereals, white flour products, rice, white potato, and processed soy products should not expect to significantly extend their life span because their diets cannot be considered nutrient-rich. The reduction in consumption of animal products is only one important feature in the design of an optimal diet, not the focal point. The critical issue for disease reduction is the nutrients-per-calorie ratio of a given diet. Unfortunately, in addition to large amounts of processed foods, vegan and vegetarian diets typically contain high amounts of added salt, which is extremely unhealthful.

You do not have to exclude all animal products from your diet to follow this plan and receive profound benefits to the health of your blood vessels and the rest of your body. You just have to reduce them to safe levels, as demonstrated in the menus and recipes in *3 Steps to Incredible Health, Volume 2*.

Humans are primates, and all other primates eat a diet of predominantly natural vegetation. While the great apes occasionally eat smaller animals, it is a very small percentage of their total caloric intake. Likewise, modern medical studies confirm that for humans to maximize their potential for a long, disease-free life, they have to keep animal product consumption to a relatively small percentage as well. Animal products are low in micronutrients, contain almost no antioxidants and phytochemicals, and are high in calories. They should be limited if you want to thrive in your later years, not just survive long enough to reproduce and then deteriorate.

In the standard American diet (SAD), less than 5 percent of the total caloric intake comes from nutrient-rich foods. This dangerously low intake of unrefined plant foods guarantees a weakened immunity from disease, leading to frequent illnesses and a shorter life span. When you eat a truly health-supporting diet, you can expect not only a drop in blood pressure and cholesterol and a reversal of heart disease, but also the elimination of headaches, constipation, indigestion, and bad breath. Achieving this means eating fewer animal products and less processed food, sugar, and flour, and eating more high-nutrient plant foods and exercising. This lifestyle shift is the key to disease protection in general.

Processed food dangers

Trans fats are extremely dangerous to the body chemistry. Trans fats are man-made fats that are used in processed foods. They are modified vegetable-derived fats that may be even worse than animal-derived saturated fats. They also are called hydrogenated oils, and they are laboratory-designed to have a similar chemical structure as saturated fat. They are solid at room temperature and have adverse health consequences. Like saturated fats, they promote heart disease and cancer.

When you are reading food labels and you see the words "partially hydrogenated" on the box, it is another way of saying trans fat, so avoid it. If you avoid processed food, it is easy to avoid trans fat. These harmful fats are found in crackers, cookies, cakes, frozen foods, and snacks.

In addition to trans fats, the baking of grains and potatoes causes browning of the food and the formation of a hard crust, which is rich in acrylamides. In the last five years, there has been worldwide alarm in the scientific community after researchers found that many of the processed foods we eat contain these cancer-causing compounds. Acrylamides form in foods that are browned by being fried, baked, roasted, grilled, or barbequed, but not in those that are steamed, boiled, or sautéed in water. Water-based cooking prevents the browning or burning that forms these harmful compounds. Frying and overcooking lead to the highest levels of acrylamides, the highest of which are found in barbequed meats, processed meats, processed cheeses, fast food meats, fried chips such as potato chips, french fries, and sugar-coated breakfast cereals.

Even though these chemicals have been shown to be potent carcinogens in animal models, so many acrylamides are consumed in the modern world that good research documenting the extent of the cancer risk in humans does not yet exist. This topic is still being actively investigated in many different countries, but the risk is difficult to estimate because baked, browned, and fried foods are so ubiquitous in Western diets.

European governments permit far fewer acrylamides in packaged foods than the United States, and they have been advising food manufacturers to reduce them. Cereals and processed foods manufactured in the United States are not under such restraints and have much higher acrylamide levels. Since the same browned and hard-baked products are rich sources of the Advanced Glycation End Products previously discussed, there are plenty of reasons to minimize or avoid these foods in your diet.

The caffeine drug

As you know, caffeine is one of the most addictive substances in a standard diet, and there is some research that indicates that excessive consumption of caffeinated beverages may pose a risk to your well-being. Coffee, however, does contain chlorogenic acid, a phenol with strong antioxidant activity that may benefit people who eat very few vegetables. So, in spite of hundreds of studies showing slightly increased risks of certain diseases such as osteoporosis and heart disease, there are also studies that show certain health benefits from coffee.[59] Either way, both the risks and the supposed benefits are marginal. One or two cups of coffee per day are not likely to cause significant disease risks.

In addition to the slightly increased risk of osteoporosis or heart disease, there are other problems with caffeine. Caffeine is a stimulant, so it gives you the false sensation that you can comfortably get by on less sleep, and inadequate sleep promotes disease and premature aging.[60] Drinking coffee also boosts estrogen levels, which worsens problems like endometriosis, breast pain, and menstrual disorders. Increased estrogen levels are also linked to higher risk of breast cancer.[61] Overall, it is difficult to discern the precise risks from heavy coffee drinking because most people who drink lots of coffee participate in lots of other unhealthful behaviors as well.

My main objection to drinking coffee is that it is addicting and, therefore, may promote more frequent eating and a higher calorie intake in some people. Eliminating your caffeine intake may help you lose weight. Coffee drinkers—and tea and cola drinkers—are drawn to eat more frequently than necessary. They eat extra meals and snacks because they mistake unpleasant caffeine withdrawal symptoms with hunger. They can't tell the difference between true hunger and the discomfort that accompanies caffeine withdrawal.

In essence, coffee is mostly like a drug, not a food. In spite of the presence of some beneficial antioxidants, it also has some negative effects and withdrawal symptoms that may fuel poor drinking and eating behavior. Like most drugs, it could have some minor benefits, but its toxic effects and resultant risks likely overwhelm those minor advantages. It is best if we aim to meet our nutritional needs with as little exposure to stimulating substances as possible. This program will work more effectively if you are able to gradually reduce and eventually eliminate coffee and other caffeine-containing substances so that you become better connected to your body's true hunger signals.

Giving detoxification a chance

It takes time to be comfortable with these changes in your life. In the process of making over your body chemistry with a healthful diet, it is not unusual to feel physically uncomfortable as you detoxify. The more stimulating or harmful your prior habits, the worse you will feel when you stop them. When breaking your addiction to salt, meat, dairy, processed foods, and other substances, you might feel headachy, fatigued, or even a little itchy or ill, but the good news is that these symptoms rarely last longer than a week or two. However, if you are making the changes to superior nutrition gradually, uncomfortable symptoms should be minimized.

Some people are so addicted to stimulating food, sugary sweets, and overeating, they may even feel depressed when they don't indulge. For example, cheese, salt, and chocolate are all addictive, and it takes a prolonged period of abstinence to beat these addictions. Sugar and caffeine, especially when mixed together, are highly addictive and create a significant amount of discomfort when eliminated from the diet. Sugar withdrawal symptoms have been demonstrated to be similar to withdrawal symptoms from opiates, including anxiety and tremors.[62] I have observed many individuals who were on drugs for severe chronic headaches and have seen them develop fever, backaches, diarrhea, and other severe detoxification symptoms after stopping medications that contain caffeine such as Excedrin, Fiorinal, and Fioricet. Fortunately, their suffering was short-lived. Through high-nutrient eating, these individuals have been able to make dramatic recoveries.

High-nutrient eating is crucial for recovery from chronic headaches or migraines. Toxic wastes build up in our tissues, and we are unable to remove them unless high levels of phytochemicals are present and the intake of toxins is stopped. These plant-based phytochemicals are necessary to enable the body's detoxification machinery. Before recovery can happen and before you can really feel your best, you must allow this detoxification to occur. An important hurdle to achieving your ideal weight and excellent health is getting rid of your addictions. After that occurs, you may feel like you have been freed from prison and will find it easier to move forward with the program. You will be one step closer to truly eating for health.

Once you learn how to prefer the most healthful foods, managing your hunger boils down to structuring your eating so that you consume the maximum number of nutrients in the fewest calories. If you consume adequate volume and nutrients, the calories will take care of themselves. The nerves lining the digestive tract send signals up to the brain, which regulates eating behavior. When our nutrient and volume needs are unfulfilled, we desire more calories to feel satisfied, and we create food addictions.

When you eat with a focus on maximizing micronutrients in relation to calories, your body function will optimize, chronic illnesses such as high blood pressure, diabetes, and high cholesterol will melt away, and you will maintain your youthful vigor into old age. You may be surprised to find that excess weight drops off at a relatively fast rate, without even trying to diet or eat less. A consistent, ideal weight is easy to maintain when nutrient needs are met with a dietary program rich in vegetables, beans, and fresh fruits. You simply don't want to overeat anymore. It's as if you had your stomach stapled, because once the micronutrient needs are met, it becomes difficult to overeat.

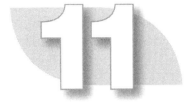

HIGH-NUTRIENT FOOD CATEGORIES

Hundreds of population studies show that raw vegetable consumption offers strong protection against cancer.[63] The National Cancer Institute recently reported on over 300 different studies that all showed the same basic information: If consumed in large enough quantities, vegetables and fruits protect against all types of cancers, and raw vegetables have the most powerful anticancer properties of all foods.[64]

Sadly, fewer than one in 100 Americans consumes enough calories from raw vegetables to ensure this defense. I encourage my patients to eat two salads each day (or have one salad plus a green smoothie or glass of freshly squeezed vegetable juice). To help you remember the importance of raw vegetables, put a big sign on your refrigerator that says, "The Salad is the Main Dish."

The word "salad" here means any vegetable eaten raw or uncooked. Fresh fruit, unsulfured dried fruits, canned beans, and a delicious dressing can be added to it. Eating a huge, delicious salad is the secret to both successful weight control and a long, healthy life.

This health-makeover program encourages you to eat raw vegetables in relatively unlimited quantities, so think big. Since they have a negative calorie effect, the more you eat, the more weight you will lose. A negative calorie effect means that the food contributes so few calories and is so bulky that it displaces space in the stomach, leading to a full feeling, which has the effect of limiting the consumption of other, more calorie-rich options. The high levels of micronutrients and fiber also help to retard appetite. Typically, you eat fewer calories at meals that feature lots of high-nutrient and calorie-negative foods. Some foods, especially raw green vegetables, supply fewer calories (even if you filled your stomach with them) than the total number of calories needed for their digestion and other important metabolic processes prior to eating again. That means that you can eat large-sized portions of these foods and still lose weight because your body will need to burn its excess fat to meet basic metabolic needs. Raw foods also have a faster transit time through the digestive tract, so all their calories are not absorbed, resulting in even more weight loss than their cooked counterparts. The objective is to eat as many raw vegetables as possible, with the goal of one pound daily. An easy way to accomplish this is to eat a salad at the beginning of your lunch, and then have some raw vegetables with a dip before dinner. This could be an entire head of lettuce with one or two tomatoes, peppers, and some shredded beets or carrots. Or, you could have cucumber and shredded cabbage with chopped apples and raisins, or raw broccoli, cherry tomatoes, and snow pea pods with a delicious humus or salsa dip. The possibilities are endless, and the menus and recipes in *3 Steps to Incredible Health, Volume 2* present many ways for you to reach this goal.

Although it may seem daunting, it is far from impossible to consume one pound of raw vegetables, especially if it is split between two meals. Believe it or not, an entire pound is less than 100 calories of food.

My longstanding advice to eat a large amount of raw vegetables (a large salad) before lunch and dinner has been tested by the medical community. Researchers used a crossover design to track the calories consumed by the same people when they ate salads as an additional first course at a meal and when they didn't. The research showed that consuming salads reduces meal-calorie intake and is an effective strategy for weight control.[65] Raw vegetables are not only for weight control; they also promote superior health in general.

When you add one of my delicious fruit, nut, or avocado-based dressings to the salad, the monounsaturated fats in the dressing increase the body's ability to absorb the anticancer compounds in the raw vegetables.[66] The synergistic combination of the raw vegetables and the healthful dressing makes the salad a health food superhero.

Greens the best

As I've discussed, all foods get their calories from fat, carbohydrate, or protein. Green vegetables, unlike high-starch vegetables like potatoes, get the majority of their calories from protein. When more of your protein needs are met from green vegetables, you get the benefit of ingesting a huge amount of critical, life-extending micronutrients.

The biggest animals all eat large amounts of green vegetation, gaining their size from the protein found there. Obviously, greens pack a powerful, nutrient-dense punch. Monkeys and apes are basically plant eaters. The greatest percentage of their daily diet comes from plant foods; they eat only small to negligible amounts of animal matter. These primates are estimated to take 95-99 percent of their diet exclusively from plant foods. The desire of these animals for a variety of plant foods in their diet supports nutrient diversity and enables them to live long lives, free of chronic diseases. The micronutrients that fuel the primate immune system are found in nature's cupboard—the garden and forest.

Humans are primates, too, and we have a very similar biology and physiology to other primates. Based on genetic information, chimpanzee and human DNA only differs by 1.6 percent. Without an adequate amount of plant-derived nutrients, we do not thrive. Our immune systems are compromised, and we develop frequent infections, allergies, autoimmune disease, and, often, cancer.

Low in calories and high in life-extending nutrients, green foods are your secret weapon to achieve incredible health. Scientific research has shown a strong positive association between the consumption of green vegetables and a reduction of all the leading causes of death in humans.[67] Cruciferous vegetables—especially broccoli, brussels sprouts, cabbage, kale, bok choy, collards, watercress, and arugula—are loaded with disease-protecting micronutrients and powerful compounds that promote detoxification and prevent cancer.

To bring your body to a phenomenal level of health, my goal is to deliver these foods to your plate in a variety of ways that make them delicious and increase your absorption of their beneficial nutrients. Greens can be served raw in salads, steamed as part of dinner, and cooked in soups and stews. When we steam or boil vegetables, some of the phytochemicals, vitamins, and minerals get lost in the water, but when we simmer vegetables in soup, all the nutrients are retained in the liquid. Additionally, the liquid base of the soup prevents the formation of toxic compounds that are created as food is browned under dry heat. Many beneficial chemical compounds are more readily absorbed when the food has been softened with heat.[68] If you have been looking through the recipes and menus in *3 Steps to Incredible Health, Volume 2*, you have found that we incorporate larger quantities of greens in an assortment of delicious ways as you move up the stages of dietary excellence.

Frozen vegetables also are a convenient option. They are picked ripe and flash-frozen right on the farm, so they are rich in micronutrients. Feel free to substitute frozen vegetables in any of your recipes.

Starchy vegetables include winter squashes, corn, potatoes, cooked carrots, sweet potatoes, yams, and pumpkins. Since they are more calorically dense than the non-starchy vegetables, they should be limited to one serving daily for those who need to lose weight. White potato is not a high-nutrient food, and many studies reveal an association between a diet high in white potato and obesity and diabetes.[69] These studies may be biased by the way potatoes are consumed (often fried or loaded with butter or sour cream), but, nevertheless, because of their relatively low nutrient density and their high glycemic index, they should play a minor role in your diet. Sweet potatoes, carrots, and peas are healthier options.

It is convenient to place whole grains, such as brown and wild rice, quinoa, millet, and whole wheat in this starchy category, but keep in mind that the colorful, high-starch vegetables, such as carrots and sweet potatoes, and black or wild rice are higher in nutrients compared to most of the grains. Whole grains are wholesome foods, but should play a smaller role in the diet as Americans eat too many grains and not enough vegetables and beans.

Fresh fruits and cancer

Fresh fruits are an important component of the natural diet of all primates. Humans and other primates have color vision and the ability to appreciate sweets. We are designed this way so that we can recognize ripe fruits and be attracted to them. We have a natural sweet tooth designed to direct us to those foods most critical for our survival.

Sugar and candy manufacturers also know that bright colors and sweet tastes are instinctually attractive. They have used that knowledge to their advantage. Remember, your instinctual reaction is designed to lead you to fruit, not sugary, processed foods. Fruit is an indispensable requirement to maintain a high level of health. Fruit consumption has been shown to offer the strongest protection against certain cancers, especially oral, esophageal, lung, prostate, and pancreatic cancer.[70]

Researchers also have discovered substances in fruit that have unique effects on preventing aging and deterioration of the brain. Some fruits, particularly berries, are rich in phytochemicals that have anti-aging effects. Berries are an excellent, nutrient-dense, low-calorie source of vitamins and phytochemicals. Researchers have seen that blueberries also have protective effects for brain health in later life.[71] In addition, certain pectins—natural parts of the cellular makeup of fruits such as oranges, kiwis, and pomegranates—also lower cholesterol and protect against cardiovascular disease.[72]

Since fruit is vital to health and well-being and can contribute to lengthening your life, I use fresh and frozen fruits to make delicious desserts that are healthful and taste great. Many delicious and easy fruit recipes are provided in 3 *Steps to Incredible Health, Volume 2* to satisfy your sweet tooth. When you complete your evening meal with one of those recipes—a frozen strawberry sorbet, a cantaloupe slush, or simply a bowl of fresh berries—you are putting the finishing touches on a meal that will satisfy your desire for a sweet food, while intellectually satisfying your desire to be healthy and wise.

You always should keep a good supply of fresh fruit on hand. It is the ultimate "convenience" food. Try to eat a variety of fruits: apples, apricots, bananas, blueberries, cherries, clementines, dates, figs, grapes, kiwis, kumquats, mangoes, melons, nectarines, oranges, papayas, peaches, pears, persimmons, pineapples, plums, pomegranates, raspberries, strawberries, and tangerines. Try some exotic fruits to add variety and interest to your diet.

If you are diabetic or on an aggressive weight-loss plan, eat more fruits that are lower in sugar, such as berries, green or Granny Smith apples, melons, oranges, kiwis, and papaya and fewer of the higher-calorie fruits such as mangoes, grapes, bananas, pineapple, and peaches. Those with diabetes do not need to avoid fruit as long as they limit it to two fresh fruits with breakfast and one with lunch and dinner. They should exclude fruit juice and eat only limited amounts of dried fruit.

Frozen fruit can be a convenient substitute when fresh fruit isn't available. The nutritional value of frozen fruit is comparable to that of fresh fruit. Avoid the canned varieties because they are not as nutritious. They often have sweeteners added and have lost most of their water-soluble nutrients.

Beans or legumes

Beans are among the world's most perfect foods. They stabilize blood sugar, blunt your desire for sweets, and prevent afternoon cravings. Beans contain both insoluble fiber and soluble fiber and are very high in resistant starch. Although resistant starch is technically a starch, it acts more like fiber and "resists" digestion. Since it passes through the small intestine undigested, it means that a significant amount of the carbohydrate calories in beans are not absorbed.

Bean intake recurs in scientific studies as an important factor promoting long life. The conclusions of an important longitudinal study show that a higher legume intake is the most protective dietary predictor of survival among the elderly, regardless of their ethnicity. The study found legumes were associated with long-lived people in various food cultures, such as the Japanese (soy, tofu, and natto), the Swedes (brown beans and peas), and the Mediterranean people (lentils, chickpeas, and white beans).[73] Beans and greens are the foods most closely linked in the scientific literature with protection against cancer, diabetes, heart disease, stroke, and dementia.

So, stock up on beans and make them your preferred high-carbohydrate food. Most of the soup and stew recipes in *3 Steps to Incredible Health, Volume 2* contain legumes. Add them to a salad to make a filling meal. Dried legumes and beans are a very economical, high-nutrient food. If you are on a food budget, use lots of dried beans in your cooking and also sprout whole beans and grains for some of your vegetable needs. Soak the whole beans in water overnight in a jar. Strain, rinse, and replace the water daily for the next few days, until the sprouts are ready to use.

If beans give you gas or bloating, make sure that you start chewing them very well. It takes some time for your digestive tract to grow the bean-digesting bacteria to digest them better. You may have to start out with a smaller quantity and increase the amount gradually. Don't stop eating beans entirely. It will make things worse when you try to eat them again. Instead, just eat a smaller amount at first, gradually increasing the amount over time.

Good fats: nuts, seeds, and avocados

High-fat plant foods are rich in the essential fatty acids that your body needs. Nuts, seeds, and avocados are some of nature's ideal foods and are the best source of healthful fats. They can satiate true hunger better than oils because they are rich in critical nutrients and fibers and have one-quarter the calories of an equal amount of oil. They should be part of your high-nutrient diet. Many people perceive raw nuts as high-fat, high-calorie foods that should be avoided or consumed in only token amounts. The important role of raw nuts and seeds in the American diet has been almost completely ignored by nutritional advisers, and their absence is a huge flaw in American cuisine. The results of recent research have changed this perception completely. Today, more and more researchers are finally aware that it is not fat in general that is the villain, but saturated fat, trans fat, and fats consumed in a processed form. Fats from avocados, raw nuts, and seeds are rich in antioxidants and phytochemicals that not only offer unique health benefits, but also maintain the freshness of the food, preventing rancidity of the fat within.

Recent evidence shows that frequent consumption of nuts is strongly protective against heart disease. An analysis of several large dietary studies found that those with the highest intake of nuts (about five times per week) had a 39 percent lower risk of coronary heart disease.[74] In addition, several clinical studies have observed beneficial effects of diets high in nuts on lowering cholesterol levels. The beneficial effects of nut consumption observed in clinical and epidemiologic studies underscore the importance of distinguishing different types of fat. One study estimated that every exchange of one ounce of saturated fat for one ounce of fat from whole nuts was associated with a 45 percent reduction in heart disease risk.[75]

Study after study shows that raw nuts and seeds not only lower cholesterol, but also extend life span and protect against common diseases of aging. They also provide a good source of protein, which makes up about 15-25 percent of their calories.[76] Raw nuts and seeds provide the most health benefits, not the salted or roasted varieties.

Over the last few years, the health benefits of seeds also have become more apparent. A tablespoon of ground flaxseed, hemp seeds, chia seeds, or other seeds can supply those hard-to-find omega-3 fats that protect against diabetes, heart disease, and cancer.[77] Seeds are also rich in lignans, a type of fiber associated with a reduced risk of both breast cancer and prostate cancer. In addition, seeds are a good source of iron, zinc, calcium, protein, potassium, magnesium, vitamin E, and folate. The plant goes to great effort in producing and protecting its seed, filling each genetic package with high concentrations of vitamins, minerals, proteins, essential oils, and enzymes.

While nuts and seeds have great health benefits, they are higher in calories and fat compared to vegetables, beans, and fruits, so they should be consumed in smaller amounts. Nuts and seeds contain about 175 calories per ounce, and a handful could be a little over one ounce. For most of us, they are not a food that should be eaten in unlimited quantity. Unless you are thin and exercising frequently, hold your consumption of raw nuts and seeds to less than two ounces per day. Many of the recipes in *3 Steps to Incredible Health, Volume 2* show how these disease-fighting foods can be used to make delicious salad dressings and dips.

Seeds, nuts, and weight loss

If you are significantly overweight and want to maximize your weight loss, you should limit your intake of seeds, nuts, and avocados to one (one-ounce) serving per day since they are calorie-rich. However, you should not exclude these healthful, high-fat foods completely from your diet. Although it may seem illogical to include such high-fat foods in your diet (since fat is nine calories a gram compared with four calories a gram for carbohydrates and protein), epidemiological studies show an inverse relationship between seed and nut consumption and body weight. Interestingly, these studies show that including some seeds and nuts in your diet actually aids in appetite suppression and weight loss. Well controlled trials that looked to see if eating nuts and seeds resulted in weight gain found the opposite; eating raw nuts and seeds promoted weight loss, not weight gain.[78]

Because seeds and nuts are rich in minerals and fiber and have a low glycemic index, they are favorable foods to include in a diet designed for diabetics and even the obese. Researchers noted that people eating one ounce of nuts five times a week reduced their risk of developing diabetes by 27 percent.[79]

There is another important reason to include nuts and seeds in your diet as you lose weight. They prevent the formation of gallstones. Weight loss in general can increase one's risk of gallstone formation, but certainly that is a reasonable risk to take when one considers the ill-health and life-threatening effects from significant body fat. It is important to note, as reported in the *American Journal of Clinical Nutrition*, that when over 80,000 women were followed for twenty years, it was found that the regular consumption of nuts and seeds offered dramatic protection against gallstone formation. These findings also have been duplicated in men.[80]

Nuts and seeds are healthful, but don't eat too many. Don't sit in front of the TV and eat an entire bag of nuts in an hour. Healthful eating means avoiding excessive calories and not eating for recreation. Nuts and seeds should be eaten with meals, not as snacks. When consumed with vegetable-containing meals, they increase absorption of the anticancer phytonutrients.

Eating to gain weight

If you are slim or want to gain weight, a larger amount of seeds, nuts, and avocados is appropriate. The amount you should consume is based on your body weight, how much fat you have on your body, and how much you exercise. A pregnant or nursing woman should consume about two ounces of seeds and nuts per day, even if overweight, and may consume more if slim. A competitive athlete may require four to six ounces or more of raw seeds and nuts per day, in addition to an avocado. In other words, some of us have a higher requirement for these higher-protein, higher-fat foods, and others need less. We do not need as much fat in our diet when we have extra fat on our body that needs to be utilized for energy, but if we are thin (and especially if your physical activity level is high), we may have a substantially higher requirement for fat and calories. Even though we need to consume a significant amount of the lower-calorie, very high-micronutrient foods, some of these higher-calorie foods are also important to fuel our caloric needs.

I provide nutritional counseling to world class and professional athletes to maximize their performance and to increase their resistance to infection. One key feature of the dietary program I recommend to them is that most of their protein and fat needs are met by consuming seeds, nuts, legumes, and avocados instead of more animal products.

I am not suggesting that these highly active individuals eat a low-fat diet. Rather, it is a diet with lots of healthful, whole food fats from seeds, nuts, and avocados. A diet with 15 percent of calories from fat could be appropriate for an overweight person with heart disease, but a slim, healthy person may find 30 percent of calories from fat is more appropriate to their needs. A highly active teenager or athlete may function best on a diet that is 40 percent or more of calories from fat. We all should consume a sufficient amount of the highest micronutrient containing super foods, but consuming seeds, nuts, and more starchy vegetables and whole grains may be necessary to meet the requirements of serious athletes with high caloric needs.

Most healthy, normal-weight individuals who exercise moderately and are in good shape can eat three to four ounces of seeds and nuts per day. That will bring their fat intake up to about 30 percent of total calories. Believing fat is the villain is wrong. For example, eating a bread, potato, and pasta-based diet is not as healthful as a diet higher in fat with fewer carbohydrate calories and more fat and protein coming from seeds and nuts. Eating more beans and whole grains can also be helpful for a person who wants to gain weight. Do not be tempted to eat more animal products to gain weight, and don't be deceived by the myth that you need a diet high in animal products to build muscles.

Whole grains

Whole grains include barley, buckwheat (kasha), millet, oats, quinoa, brown rice, and wild rice, all of which are high in fiber. Just because a food is called "whole grain" doesn't mean that it is a good food. Many whole grain cold cereals are so processed that they do not have a significant fiber per serving ratio and have lost most of their nutritional value. The intact (unground) whole grains and the more coarsely ground grains are absorbed into the bloodstream more slowly. They are more healthful, and they curtail appetite more effectively.

As you know by now, to eat healthfully, fruits and vegetables should form the base of your food pyramid. That means that grains should be consumed in a much smaller amount than you were probably eating before. Grains simply do not contain enough nutrients per calorie to form a substantial part of your diet. You will notice that as you move from Level 1 to Level 2 to Level 3 of my menu plans, grain products are gradually reduced.

Many scientific studies show a strong association between the consumption of white flour products, such as pasta and bread, with diabetes, obesity, and heart disease.[81] Refined carbohydrates also are linked to enlargement of the prostate.[82] These results continue to show that eating white flour and sweeteners is nutritional suicide.

Whole grains are the least nutrient-dense foods of the seed family and they do not show the powerful protection against disease that is apparent in the scientific studies of fresh fruit, vegetables, beans, raw nuts, or seeds. Sprouted grains and grains cooked in water are healthier and more nutritious to eat than precooked breakfast cereals. Some of the healthier grains to consume include hulled barley, buckwheat (kasha), millet, oats, quinoa, and wild rice. As a minor part of your diet, they can be water-cooked and used as a breakfast cereal with fruits and nuts or as a dinner side dish.

Animal products

As you move through this program, the goal is to limit animal products to 10 percent of caloric intake or less. On the days when you do include animal products in a meal, limit the serving size to under four ounces. Do not make animal products the focus of the meal. Think of them as a garnish, condiment, or flavoring agent.

The Level 1 meal plan permits more animal products than I generally recommend. It still is a large reduction in animal product intake for most people and an important first step. If you are comfortable eating fewer animal products in Level 1, go for it. Full-fat dairy, such as cheese and butter, are the foods with the highest saturated fat content, so choose fat-free dairy products, and for the same reason, try to choose white meat fowl, fish, and eggs. Avoid processed meats, barbecued meats, luncheon meats, bacon, hot dogs, and any pickled, darkened, blackened, barbecued, or overcooked animal products.

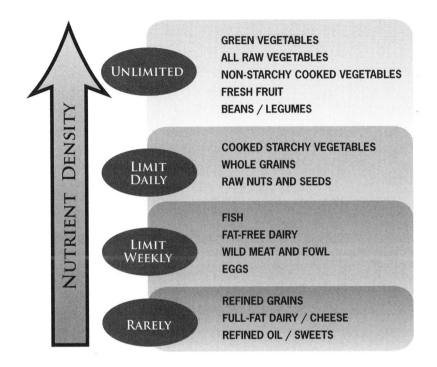

NUTRIENT DENSITY

UNLIMITED
GREEN VEGETABLES
ALL RAW VEGETABLES
NON-STARCHY COOKED VEGETABLES
FRESH FRUIT
BEANS / LEGUMES

LIMIT DAILY
COOKED STARCHY VEGETABLES
WHOLE GRAINS
RAW NUTS AND SEEDS

LIMIT WEEKLY
FISH
FAT-FREE DAIRY
WILD MEAT AND FOWL
EGGS

RARELY
REFINED GRAINS
FULL-FAT DAIRY / CHEESE
REFINED OIL / SWEETS

Keep in mind that eating to maintain extra fat stores on your body, because you or others think you look better heavier, is never healthful. A healthy person is slim and muscular. If you think you are too thin and desire more weight on your frame, the right way to achieve that is from working out in the gym, not in the kitchen. The muscular demands on your body will then increase your appetite, hunger will occur more frequently, and your caloric intake will increase proportionally to the increased muscular demand. If you want to gain weight, try to make your thighs, shoulders, and chest a little bigger with more exercise. Don't expand your waistline by over-exercising your knife and fork.

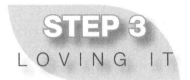

STEP 3
LOVING IT

SUPER FOODS, SUPER HEALTH AND THE PLEASURE OF EATING

Before we take *Step 3* and start learning about Super Foods, Super Health and the Pleasure of Eating, let's take a look at the last success stories in this book. (If you'd like to read more, you will find plenty more of them at www.DrFuhrman.com, along with many other support materials.)

From your reading so far, it will be clear that the power of superior nutrition is what you need to reach your weight and health goals. Don't underestimate the happiness and enjoyment of life changes that also will occur. After all, that is what health ultimately is about.

I hope that you already are reaping benefits from your increasingly better dietary practices and that these initial successes will inspire you to pursue even greater ones as time goes on.

CARLA — ASTHMA, ALLERGIES, AND LUPUS

I was a healthy, active kid and adolescent; however, in my late teens and early twenties, I developed multiple health issues. Over time, my symptoms accumulated in the following order: exercise-induced asthma, environmental allergies, Raynaud's phenomenon, chilblains (sores on my fingers and toes accompanied by terrible swelling, pain, and arthritis), hip problems, daily headaches and migraines, terrible neck pain, mouth ulcers, sore throats and chronic infections, an episode of mononeucleosis, body aches, muscle and joint pain, debilitating fatigue, and thinning hair. I think you will agree that I was experiencing a very poor quality of life.

About six years into this downward spiral, I received confirmation that I was dealing with a connective tissue disease, probably mild lupus, and given the standard medications. At that point, I was already on multiple prescription medications and nutritional supplements. I was absolutely miserable and barely making it through my workdays. Eventually, at the age of twenty-seven, I was forced to stop working altogether. When I researched lupus, I only found drug therapies—no other options, which gave me little hope. The medication I was taking thinned my once-thick hair. It also made me lose my appetite, my appreciation for life, and the ability to do the simplest of tasks. I had transformed from a young, healthy, and active individual into a sick, suffering existence that I was unwilling to accept. Despite what I was told, I knew that I did not want to be on medications for the rest of my life, and I vowed that eventually I would become healthy again.

A year after my diagnosis, I learned about Dr. Fuhrman, read his book, and shortly after that made an appointment to see him. With each passing month, I feel more and more like my former, productive self. I am thrilled to have my life back. I'm off all medications except Allegra, as needed (which I plan to get off completely.) My energy levels are much improved, and my overall pain has decreased dramatically. I exercise most days of the week, and can run for four miles. I am working full-time again, and I have a renewed appreciation for being pain- and inflammation-free. My sedimentation rate (inflammatory marker) has dropped from 25 down to 2, my ssDNA (lupus marker) has dropped from 130 to 66, and my total cholesterol has dropped from 198 to 119.

I still get run-down at times and occasionally experience mild symptoms, but overall my quality of life has improved substantially. For the first time in a long time, I feel like I can have a normal life again. Best of all, I have great faith that I will continue to improve over time and become healthier with each passing year. I have regained control of my health destiny and am deeply thankful to Dr. Fuhrman, his family, and his entire staff for all of their sacrifice and help. High-nutrient eating has ended my suffering, restored my health, and enriched my life, both personally and professionally.

Tom — Diabetes and Obesity

I have been a Type II diabetic for more than twenty years, using Humolog and Lantus, as well as being morbidly obese, weighing 338 pounds. I had tried to lose weight previously, but was unsuccessful. However, after reading Dr. Fuhrman's book, I thought I would try again, following his high-nutrient program.

Currently, I am in my seventh week of the program. I have lost 40 pounds, stopped using insulin, have an average glucometer reading of 97, and an A1C of 5.8. I have renewed energy, my leg and foot pain is gone, and I haven't had an asthma attack in seven weeks. I feel great. Dr. Fuhrman has given me back my life.

TRISHA — FAMILY WEIGHT LOSS

The first day I started Dr. Fuhrman's program I felt different—I had more energy. Soon, I began to crave leafy greens like never before. My health improved, I lost weight, and I felt happier than I had in a long time. I even lost weight over the Thanksgiving holiday (no small feat in my very Southern family). I feel great knowing that I'm feeding my family better, and I don't crave food when my emotions swing. My sweet husband also has started this program, and he has lost 25 pounds. Best of all, after only four weeks on the program, he is off all of his blood pressure medication.

HAROLD — DIABETES, HIGH BLOOD PRESSURE, AND HIGH CHOLESTEROL

Before I read Dr. Fuhrman's *Eat to Live*, I was diagnosed with Type II diabetes. I was running to the bathroom every twenty minutes. I went to a walk-in medical clinic and learned that I had a blood glucose level of 458, high blood pressure, and high cholesterol. I was put on three medications initially, and then another when the blood glucose level didn't come down enough. My business was suffering because I had no inspiration, no desire, and no energy. I was considering selling my musical instruments to pay for my medications and my eventual deathbed. And I was only forty-five years old.

Fortunately, I had purchased *Eat to Live* two years prior. Unfortunately, I hadn't read it. In desperation, I pulled it off the shelf and started reading. I soon felt a psycho-spiritual-physical shift, before I even finished reading it. I felt as though someone was throwing me a last-minute lifeline. I started following the program immediately—no hesitation, no thinking about it, just action. Within two and a half weeks, I was off all my medication. No Glucophage, no Glipizide, no Linsinipril, no Lipitor. As the pounds started to disappear, a renewed sense of self-esteem began to reappear, and with this came renewed vitality. Joy was returning to my life!

Within four months, I was 90 pounds lighter, I started exercising again, and I felt completely transformed. It's incredible, and this is just the beginning for me. My restored health and love of life are something I will be forever grateful for.

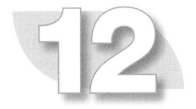

EXERCISES WITH FOOD:
THE ADVANCED WORKOUT

At this point, we are about to take *Step 3*, and learn about Super Foods, Super Health and the Pleasure of Eating. To help accelerate the process, it's time for some advanced exercises. As you already know from the previous ones that you have been doing, Exercises with Food can help increase the pleasure you derive from natural food, which will help you adjust to eating with the goal of superior nutrition. Like all exercises, they require frequent practice in order to see results. Continue doing the previous exercises with a particular focus on stretching the palate. This will help you rid yourself of toxic hunger.

Here are three advanced exercises for you.

EXERCISE 5

Make a point to eat a light lunch or a light breakfast each day. Eating one lighter meal without snacking before the next meal, either lunch or dinner, will increase your true hunger before that meal. Over time, this will help to teach you what true hunger feels like. The main exercise target here is to see if you can get back in touch with sensations of "true hunger," differentiating the sensation from "toxic hunger." Be patient because it may take some time for toxic hunger to go away. It will help if you link together an entire week of superior nutrition so that you can lose the toxic hunger symptoms and begin the pleasurable sensation of true hunger.

EXERCISE 6

Reduce your consumption of animal products (meat, eggs, and dairy products) to no more than one serving per day, with an eventual goal of eating no more than one serving per week. Use the high-nutrient recipes in *3 Steps to Incredible Health, Volume 2* to replace animal products in your menus.

EXERCISE 7

Remove white flour, sugar, and other sweeteners from your diet. This means using fewer processed foods. Store-purchased products should be 100 percent whole grain and contain no sweetening agents.

Adopting the high-nutrient diet is a big change for most people, but clearly it is not an all-or-nothing plan. It is a journey toward taking control of your own health destiny. No matter what phase or level you start with, positive changes will provide rewards. Have fun, enjoy your food, and eat for health.

Workout Performance Goals

- Continue doing the exercises from previous chapters.

- Eat a light breakfast or lunch and learn to experience the feeling of "true" hunger.

- Greatly reduce the amount of animal products (meat, fish, and dairy products) in your diet.

- Eliminate or greatly reduce refined, processed foods made with white sugar and white flour.

How will I be different two years from now?

Today's date _____

Two years from now:

_____

_____

_____

_____

_____

_____

_____

_____

_____

_____

_____

_____

_____

_____

_____

_____

_____

_____

_____

_____

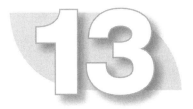

THREE COMPONENTS OF HEALTH

If you felt compelled to begin this journey, it was likely instinct that was driving you. Every living organism has a built-in instinct to survive and to thrive. As you continue on the path towards maximizing your health, you will reach the point where this type of nutrient-rich eating will become second nature. By being consistent in putting your newly obtained knowledge into practice, it will become ingrained as your healthful, new way of living. If you have been doing the food exercises I have recommended, you are probably already feeling a lot better than before and have the desire to feel even better.

In the next few chapters, I will be giving you additional information to further your path to great health. Many people invest in their financial future, but never consider their health future. The way you take care of yourself is just as crucial a determinant of your future happiness as your savings account. A large nest egg is of no use to you if you're not there to spend it!

As you plan for your health future, you must consider the three important components that pay you back with high returns: your nutritional, physical, and social states. Each factor must be considered.

- **Nutritional component**—Make every calorie count as you strive for maximum nutrition. Remember my health equation, H = N/C. Strive to eat foods that have high nutrient-density scores.

- **Physical component**—Make physical exercise a part of your normal routine. Joining a gym is a great bonus, but learn to exploit all of the other opportunities in your life to exercise your body during the normal course of the day. Take the stairs instead of the elevator. When possible, walk instead of riding. Once you embrace my high-nutrient diet, you can strive for physical excellence. You may find that exercise becomes easier and more pleasurable with better health and a lower weight.

- **Social component**—Build a strong mental defense against unhealthful influences. A healthy mindset is a prerequisite for a healthy lifestyle, and the best way to develop it is to be optimistic and surround yourself with people who engage in and support your health. Even if you don't feel naturally optimistic, you can learn the attitude. Just reading this book shows that you are optimistic.

These three factors are all healthful habits that will eventually become second nature. The more you do them, the more they become your preferred way of life. Many unhealthy and healthy people are obsessed with food. Eating the right foods will make you incredibly healthy, but avoid obsessions even with healthful foods. They are often indicators of compulsions and other social and psychological issues.

Striking a balance between eating and not eating is an excellent way to eliminate the obsession and strive for a fully balanced life where people, food, pleasure, recreation, exercise, work, rest, and sleep all have their place. The key to finding food's place in this balance is making the material you're learning instinctive and a natural part of your life.

Addictions make attempts at dietary modifications more difficult, but it only takes a few seconds of decision-making to win the battle and say an emphatic "no" to the addiction and "yes" to your new healthful lifestyle. I want to mention again that I have observed thousands of cases in which these positive changes have resulted in some temporary discomfort, while the body eliminates toxins and restores its cells to a more youthful, decongested state. This is normal, and coping with it on the road to better health will be a small price to pay. By now, some change has certainly occurred in your life as a result of learning this body of knowledge and beginning to eat a nutrient-dense diet.

Do not underestimate the human body's powerful capacity for self-healing when superior nutrition has been established and dietary and emotional stresses have been removed. Many people have made these changes and have completely recovered from chronic illnesses that their doctors told them they would have forever.

During most of human history, getting adequate calories was a difficult struggle. In those days, malnutrition from food scarcity was the major problem, not obesity. Humans are able to survive in so many environments because we are the most adaptable species on the planet. Now, our adaptability has become a liability because unhealthful options have become so accessible. However, you can control the choices that you make. This book is about change and restoration. Hopefully, it will spur you to confront your fears about different dietary choices, reclaim your natural tastes, and restore your natural hunger drive.

Stubborn habits

You've learned which foods are best for your body, and you've been practicing high-nutrient eating (ideally with the help of the menus and recipes in *3 Steps to Incredible Health, Volume 2,*) so you know that you can eat most healthful foods to your heart's content. It sounds like all your food problems are solved. Or are they? Do you still crave unhealthful foods and eat even when you aren't hungry? Let's talk briefly again about food addictions and how to get beyond them.

Modern foods are designed to seduce your taste buds. You have been manipulated by profit-motivated food manufacturers. We all have. The artificially concentrated flavors that the processed food industry uses to stimulate the brain's pleasure center are designed to increase and retain sales. Processed and refined foods entice us to eat even when we are not truly hungry. Tragically, the result is that they lead people's taste buds astray. Artificial, intense flavors cause us to enjoy natural flavors less. We become desensitized, and the more we succumb to the heightened, artificial flavors, the less appealing natural, whole foods become. As we have discussed, salt also overwhelms our taste buds. We need more and more to experience any pleasurable sensation.

Fortunately, by practicing the high-nutrient diet, your sensory abilities will start bouncing back. It may take time to reset your receptors to appreciate the more subtle flavors of whole, unprocessed foods. Hang in there, and keep up your healthful eating! It's the only way for this to happen, and it always does. It might take longer than six weeks, but your taste and flavor sensitivity will improve tremendously over time.

Realizing your impediments and gaining knowledge about great health are tremendous first steps, but they are only half of the overall solution. You must put into practice and repeat your new beneficial behaviors over and over until they become part of you. Repetition will make these positive actions feel more and more natural. The more you make healthful meals, and the more days you link together eating healthful foods, the more your brain will naturally prefer to eat this way.

Developing a burning desire for optimal health will help you in this process. Stay with the program, and your taste buds will line up with your desires, your behaviors will line up with your beliefs, and you will cease to crave flavor enhancers and highly seasoned food. You will transform into a person who actually prefers to eat healthfully. As you learn more recipes, you will be able to substitute similar, healthful foods for those old, unhealthful ones. For example, the healthful sorbets and "ice creams" in *3 Steps to Incredible Health, Volume 2* are the perfect substitute for your craving of cold sweets.

It is not easy to develop new habits, and there is no such thing as a quick shortcut to developing new skills and expertise. However, if you are motivated to persevere and keep trying, the change becomes considerably easier. Feeling better and losing weight are great motivators. Don't give up. The only failure is to stop trying.

Planning and exercise

The ability to consistently make good decisions requires good planning. You need time to prepare your environment so that you have good-tasting, healthful foods around you at all times to minimize temptation. Because eating healthfully has only gained popularity in recent years, few restaurants or fast-food places make eating this way convenient. And because most of us work, it can be tough to fit everything, including cooking and exercise, into our busy schedules. Therefore, if you are going to succeed at turning your health or weight around, you will need to organize your time.

This book is not about exercise, but it is still important to mention it. Without regular exercise, you cannot expect to secure great health benefits. For excellent health in our later years, excellent nutrition must go hand in hand with regular, vigorous exercise. Our muscles and bones will shrink and weaken as we age if we do not exercise regularly and place demands on our skeleton. Osteoporosis is mostly the result of a sedentary lifestyle.

If you shop and cook twice each week, you can still have time to exercise on the other days. Plenty of people exercise four times per week by following a schedule such as this: Exercise once on Saturday, once on Sunday, and then two more times during the week. Below is a sample of a schedule of eating plans and exercising that you can modify for your own needs.

Saturday	Eat out, salad bar, or take-out food	Exercise A
Sunday	Shop and cook	Exercise B
Monday	Eat leftovers	day off
Tuesday	Eat leftovers	Exercise A
Wednesday	Shop and cook	day off
Thursday	Eat leftovers	Exercise B
Friday	Eat leftovers	day off

Exercise A days:

Walk uphill on an incline treadmill, skip rope, or ride a bike; plus work out your abs, lower back, and chest. Even fifteen minutes of heartbeat-elevating, calorie-burning cardio, such as walking on a steep incline or pedaling on an elliptical machine, is good. If using a treadmill, gradually increase the incline as your cardiovascular fitness and exercise tolerance improves.

Exercise B days:

Exercise on an elliptical machine or a stair-climber; plus work out legs, biceps, triceps, latissimus dorsi, and trapezius with weights or resistance. Aim for some cardio activities with an elevated pulse four times each week.

Make a list of all the exercises that you like to do and separate them into two different workouts. For example, make the A exercise day easier on the thighs and the B exercise day heavier on the thighs so that you will be able to handle the B exercise day, even if it is the next day, without having your legs feel too tired.

Your exercise schedule and what exercises or activities you do should be individualized to your needs and preferences. The underlying theme is to plan it into your schedule. Do not exercise the same body parts on consecutive days, and spread out many different exercises to encompass various body parts into your weekly plan. If you are new to exercise, start slowly so you do not injure yourself. Begin by walking on a treadmill with only a three to four degree incline and lifting some very light dumbbells. Over time, keep increasing the incline on the treadmill, so you can eventually perform a more vigorous workout and burn more calories in your time allotment. Only increase speed on the treadmill after your increasing fitness level has enabled you to perform comfortably at the highest incline. It is better to go slower at a higher incline than to go faster at a lower incline. It puts less stress on your joints, and you burn more calories.

If you belong to a fitness facility or have access to a fitness professional, inquire about other exercises and the proper form of your workouts. Don't push yourself too hard, but make sure that you are doing physical exercise at least three times per week.

If you are significantly overweight, diabetic, or have heart disease, and your capacity for vigorous exercise is low, you will need to exercise more frequently, even two or three times per day. The lower your fitness level and the lower the intensity of exercise that you are capable of, the more frequently you need to exercise. Many of my patients with diabetes exercise twice daily. It is like their medicine before lunch and dinner. Even ten minutes of exercise, done regularly, is better than no exercise.

The more thoroughly you plan your weekly schedule in advance, the easier it will be to ingrain your new habits into your life. We live busy lives, we work hard, and we have to plan even our recreational activities and vacations in advance. So, make a weekly health plan and figure out:

- When are you going to shop?

- What are you going to purchase when you shop? (Be sure to make a list!)

- What dishes, soups, or dressings are you going to prepare when you cook?

- What dishes are you going to make in large volume for use on multiple days and store in the refrigerator or freezer?

- What frozen vegetables and fruits are you going to have on hand?

- When are you going to exercise?

- What exercises or activities are you going to do?

- When will you go to sleep and wake up?

- How many relaxation, entertainment, and social activities can you plan to fit in?

Remember, not only does regular exercise burn calories during the time you are actually exercising, it also increases the caloric needs of your body into the days ahead, even on the days you are not exercising. It will work with your new diet to deliver dramatic benefits. Exercise is the only way to increase your metabolic rate, healthfully.

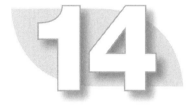

SNACKING, SHOPPING, AND EATING OUT

Most people agree that they make better food choices if they make a point of eliminating temptations. It is best if you can get rid of all the unhealthful food in your kitchen. If it isn't in the house, you won't be faced with the constant question of whether or not to eat it. Instead, stock up on nutrient-rich, healthful foods. This strategy can be one of the most important steps toward healthful living. Eventually, healthful food will taste just as good as unhealthful options. You just have to learn the best ways to prepare it and how to get your taste buds in shape to enjoy it.

If your family does not want to join your health makeover, then create a separate area in the pantry and refrigerator for your foods. It is more challenging if you have to make unhealthful foods for your family while you're in the midst of your own health makeover, but don't let the obstacles stop you. Remember, by making yourself healthier and enjoying it, you are opening the door for others to potentially follow your lead. Share what you are learning and your excitement about your changes, and let each person come to their own conclusions in their own time. It is very likely that when your family and friends see you looking and feeling better, they will want to know more about what you are doing, and you will eventually have others join you on your quest for better health.

To snack or not to snack

For maximum success, it is best to eat only when you are hungry and to stop eating as soon as you feel satisfied. This will require less will-power as you progress and get better at meeting your body's nutritional and volume requirements. I want you to try to get back in touch with your body's signals. Try to eat only when you feel hungry, and as time progresses, pay attention to see if you can develop the ability to distinguish true hunger—felt in the throat—from the symptoms of toxic hunger. Remember, the symptoms of toxic hunger, which are caused by withdrawal, won't turn off until you have provided your body with adequate nutrients and your body has had time to build up a nutrient reserve in its tissues. This could take a few weeks to a few months, so be patient.

Eating when hungry usually translates into a three-meal-per-day format, without snacking. Many people do fine on two meals per day, too. Unless you are a dedicated athlete or a physical laborer, you probably don't burn enough calories to justify snacking. Snacking is most often recreational eating, without true hunger present. It has negative effects, including the following:

- usually results in the consumption of a higher amount of calories each week

- prevents you from experiencing true hunger before meals, thus diminishing enjoyment of food

- prevents your digestive tract from getting the rest it needs to build up digestive enzymes for proper digestion.

- detoxification and cellular repair progress less efficiently

Animal studies have shown that eating less frequently results in increased life span. The healthier you eat, the quicker the desire to eat between meals and the symptoms of toxic hunger will disappear.

Some helpful hints to combat snacking are:

- Eat a salad or raw vegetables with a dip to start both lunch and dinner.

- Keep lots of frozen fruits and vegetables and prewashed fresh foods in your home.

- Have cooked greens or soups with greens at every lunch and dinner.

- Don't eat after 8:00 p.m.

- Have a fruit sorbet or fruit dessert after dinner, and then clean the kitchen, clean your teeth, and end eating for the day.

Food shopping

Your health makeover will require some brushing up on your shopping skills. It's easy to shop for high-nutrient foods; they are mostly in the produce aisle. Since it is necessary to consume a variety of fresh fruits and vegetables, I recommend that you shop twice a week. You will use the main shopping trip of the week to stock up on staples and produce for three or four days. Your second trip of the week can be a short trip to restock fresh fruits and vegetables. You will spend most of your time in the produce, health food, and frozen food sections. The supermarket is filled with temptation, so try to avoid certain aisles. The center aisles of most stores contain the most heavily processed foods; consider them nonexistent and do not travel down those aisles. What you don't see can't tempt you!

You can use all spices and herbs except for salt. When using condiments, mustard is okay if unsalted mustard is available, but pickled foods typically contain too much salt and should be avoided. If you love ketchup or tomato sauce, you may find a lower calorie, low-salt ketchup and tomato sauce at the health food store.

Food labels

I want you to read food labels, but you'll get the best dietary outcomes if you try to avoid foods that have labels. With the exception of unprocessed frozen fruits or vegetables, foods that come in boxes, bags, and jars are usually highly processed and low in nutrients-per-calorie. When you buy foods that have labels, be selective and use good judgment. If you know what to look for and how to interpret it, food labels can help you evaluate the healthfulness of a product. Don't be misled by the other writing on the package. It is essentially advertising, and tells you little, if anything, about the nutritional content of the product. The ingredient list contains the most important information. It is often in very small print and difficult to find and read, but read it you must. Inspect the label before you add an item to your shopping cart.

Reading labels reinforces the idea that you need to put some products back on the shelf. Avoid foods that list white flour (often called wheat flour) and any type of sweetener, such as corn syrup, among the first few ingredients. Ingredients are listed on the label according to quantity, in descending order based on weight (from most to least). As a general rule of thumb, if the list of ingredients is long and you cannot pronounce most of them, there are probably a lot of chemical additives in the product, and you're risking your health by eating it.

Be sure to read the ingredients even when purchasing foods from a health food store or when the rest of the packaging is trying to convince you the food is healthful. For example, watch out for statements like these on packages:

- natural fruit flavors

- with real fruit juice

- all natural ingredients

- no artificial preservatives

- 100% natural

- real fruit

- no preservatives

- no artificial ingredients

Statements like these do not mean that there are no harmful additives in the product or that the products are healthful. They simply mean the manufacturer hopes you'll think there are no harmful ingredients. For example, here is the list of ingredients from a loaf of bread that claims "ALL NATURAL INGREDIENTS" and "NO ARTIFICIAL PRESERVATIVES ADDED" on its label:

Enriched wheat flour (wheat flour, malted barley, niacin, reduced iron, thiamine mononitrate, riboflavin), water, high fructose corn syrup, yeast, wheat bran, vital wheat gluten, butter. Contains 2 percent or less of each of the following: rye meal, corn flour, molasses, rolled whole wheat, salt, dough conditioners (ammonium sulfate, sodium stearoyl lactylate), brown sugar, honey, vinegar, oatmeal, soy flour, mono and diglycerides, partially hydrogenated soybean oil.

As you read this list, notice that the first two ingredients are white flour and sugar. This bread is junk food.

- Enriched wheat flour is white flour. The bran and the germ portion of the whole wheat, which are rich in vitamins and minerals, have been removed. To compensate for refining out approximately twenty nutrients, four are added back. Use only whole wheat flour; it must have the word "whole" on the label.

- High fructose corn syrup is a concentrated form of sugar derived from corn.

- Dough conditioners, in general, can cause mineral deficiencies, and ammonium sulfate in particular may cause mouth ulcers, nausea, and kidney and liver problems.

- Brown sugar is merely white sugar with molasses added.

- Partially hydrogenated soybean oil is a trans fat associated with heart disease, breast and colon cancer, atherosclerosis, and elevated cholesterol. It is even worse than saturated fat.

As you can see, this "all-natural" bread will not help you on your road to health. Even if you didn't know the particular detriments of each ingredient, taking the time to read that its main ingredients are white flour and sugar, and that the rest of the list is lengthy, would tell you to leave it on the shelf.

When looking at labels, we also need to be aware of sodium levels. A lot of sodium is "hidden" in processed foods, from spaghetti sauce to canned soup to frozen dinners. Obviously, if you see the word "salt" on a food label, you know salt is in the product. But baking soda and monosodium glutamate (MSG) contain sodium, too. To avoid excess sodium, try to avoid products with: brine, disodium phosphate, garlic salt, onion salt, sodium alginate, sodium benzoate, sodium caseinate, sodium citrate, sodium hydroxide, sodium nitrate, sodium pectinate, sodium proprionate, and sodium sulfite. Also avoid anything using the words "pickled," "cured," "broth," and "soy sauce." They all indicate high sodium.

Just because a product says that it has reduced sodium or is light in sodium does not mean it is a low-salt product. It only means it has less than the higher-salt version of the product. Lots of these products still contain far too much salt for good health.

IF THE LABEL SAYS...	IT MEANS...
sodium-free/salt-free	less than 5 mg sodium per serving
very low-sodium	less than 35 mg sodium per serving
low-sodium	less than 140 mg sodium per serving
reduced sodium	at least 25% less sodium than original product
light in sodium	at least 50% less sodium than original product
unsalted/no added salt	no salt added during processing (not necessarily sodium-free)

You want to keep your overall daily sodium intake under 1200 mg and preferably under 1000 mg. Natural foods contain less than 0.5 mg of sodium per calorie. If a serving of food provides 100 calories and it contains 400 mg of sodium, then you know it has had plenty of salt added to it. Since you get 400-700 mg of sodium daily from natural whole foods, you don't want processed foods to push you over the limit. Be sure to read the food labels, and do not add more than 200-400 mg of extra sodium per day, so you don't push yourself up over that 1000-1200 mg limit.

In addition to sodium, most processed foods contain a litany of food additives with toxic properties. Substances such as artificial colors, sweeteners, stabilizers, nitrates, and preservatives often are linked to cancer in lab animals and may be harmful or cancer-promoting in humans. They are best avoided.

- Food labels list ingredients in decreasing order. What's first on the ingredient list is present in the highest quantity.

- Do not purchase foods that contain white flour (also written as wheat flour) or sweeteners in the first four ingredients or that contain any hydrogenated (trans) fat or chemical additives.

- Avoid foods with more mg of sodium than the amount of calories in the serving size.

Eating in restaurants

Dining out can be challenging when transitioning to a high-nutrient diet. The first step when going out to eat is to find a restaurant that will have some healthful options. Many restaurants will cater to your needs and preferences. Call ahead and ask. Eat early before the restaurant gets very crowded so the staff will have time to modify a dish or make something for you.

If your restaurant meal is a breakfast, stay away from the bread, bagels, and breakfast sweets. It is easy to find oatmeal, fruit, or eggs.

For lunch and dinner, ask for an extra side order of steamed vegetables instead of pasta or white rice to accompany your main dish. Patronize restaurants that have salad bars. You also can order Asian vegetable dishes that are steamed or water sautéed with the dressing or sauce on the side. Because soups are made in advance in restaurants and are always very high in salt, it is best that you do not eat soups when you are out. Stick with salads and a main dish. I often order a double-sized salad and let them charge me double. I often will order a double-sized portion of whatever green vegetable they have fresh, adding, "Can you make that without oil, salt, or butter?" Then I add the vegetables to my salad.

Ask the waiter not to bring bread to the table, so you are not tempted to fill up before the meal. Always order the salad dressing on the side so you can use their high-salt dressings sparingly. You also can ask if they have olive oil to use instead of butter on potatoes or to use (with or without vinegar) instead of the high-salt salad dressing.

The more you practice, the better you will get at handling all of the many eating situations that arise. Remember, the goal is not to eat perfectly at every single meal. The goal is to eat very well the vast majority of the time. If you eat an unhealthful meal, don't despair; just start eating healthfully again at your next meal.

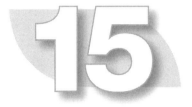

THREE STEPS TO INCREDIBLE HEALTH

The practical application of my high-nutrient program centers around the three-level menu plans. In *3 Steps to Incredible Health, Volume 2*, I have designed the three levels for you. All you need to do is pick a level and get started. I am going to describe the three levels here as well, so that you can start to envision the right level for you and start to devise your own menus.

Menu levels

Based on your health needs and current dietary habits, you can choose between three different levels of superior nutrition, starting on Level 1 and working your way up to Level 3. I would like to see everyone reach at least Level 2, although for many people, even Level 1 represents a significant improvement.

Over time, as your taste and food preferences change and you become more comfortable eating high-nutrient foods, consider moving to a higher level. Keep your focus on increasing your intake of disease-protective nutrients by eating whole natural foods. Use my scoring system, *Dr. Fuhrman's Nutrient Density Scores*, in Chapter 3 to help you choose more of the most nutrient-dense foods. When you eat foods with very high scores, you will be satisfied with fewer calories and less likely to overeat.

As you design your menus, keep in mind that the menus in *3 Steps to Incredible Health, Volume 2* provide approximately 1400 calories daily. For most people, this will result in moderate weight loss. If you do not need to lose weight, you can include some of the options listed at the bottom of each day's menu or include a more generous amount of raw nuts and seeds in your diet. Because this is not a calorie-counting diet, you can eat as much as you desire. When you eat a micronutrient-rich diet, you naturally desire fewer calories. Everyone has different caloric needs, so you may require more or fewer calories than suggested in the menus. Eat when you are hungry. If you are not hungry, don't eat.

Menu guidelines

Use the following high-nutrient guidelines as you design your individual menus.

FOR ALL LEVELS, INCLUDE DAILY:

1) a large salad

2) at least a half-cup serving of beans/legumes in soup, salad, or some other dish

3) at least three fresh fruits

4) at least one ounce of raw nuts and seeds

5) at least one large (double-sized) serving of steamed green vegetables

AVOID:

1) barbequed, processed, and cured meats and red meat

2) fried foods

3) full-fat dairy (cheese, ice cream, butter, whole milk, and two percent milk), and trans fat (margarine)

4) soft drinks, sugar, and artificial sweeteners

5) white flour products

Level 1 is appropriate for a person who is healthy, thin, physically fit, and exercises regularly. You should have no risk factors such as high blood pressure, high cholesterol, or a family history of heart disease, stroke, or cancer before age 75.

Most Americans do have risk factors or a family history of strokes, heart attacks, and cancer, and most Americans are overweight. So most people should only see Level 1 as a temporary stage as they learn about high-nutrient eating and allow their taste buds to acclimate to whole, natural plant foods.

Level 1 is designed to ease the emotional shock of making profound dietary improvements. It enables people to revamp their diet at a level that is significant, but not overwhelming. Enjoy this new style of eating, allow your taste preferences to change with time, and learn some great recipes. You soon may decide to move up to a higher level. However, I still recommend that the majority of individuals make the commitment to jump right into the more nutrient-dense Levels 2 and 3 because so many people are significantly overweight and have risk factors that need to be addressed immediately. People in desperate need of a health makeover need to start on Levels 2 or 3.

On Level 1, you eliminate fried foods and substitute fruit-based healthful desserts and whole grains for low-nutrient processed snack foods such as salty snacks, candy, ice cream, and baked products. Whole grain products like old-fashioned oats, wild rice, brown rice, 100 percent whole grain bread, and pasta made with 100 percent whole grain or bean flour are used. Bread and pasta made with white flour are eliminated.

Your sodium intake will decrease as you begin to make these dietary changes. Processed foods and restaurant foods contribute 77 percent of the sodium people consume. Salt from the saltshaker provides 11 percent, and sodium found naturally in food provides the remaining 12 percent.

You also eliminate foods like cheese and butter that are high in saturated fats. Your cooking techniques use no oil, or only occasional use of a minimal amount of oil. Most Americans consume over fifteen servings of animal products weekly. On Level 1, I recommend only four servings of animal products per week. These animal products are limited to fish, chicken, turkey, eggs, or grass-fed organic dairy and meats.

LEVEL 2 GUIDELINES

Level 2 builds on the positive changes described for Level 1. On Level 2, animal products are reduced to three servings weekly, and vegetables and beans make up an even larger portion of your total caloric intake. When you incorporate more and more nutrient-rich produce in your diet, you automatically increase your intake of antioxidants, phytochemicals, plant fibers, lignins, and plant sterols. You lower the glycemic index of your diet and the level of saturated fat, salt, and other negative elements without having to think about it. Your ability to appreciate the natural flavors of unprocessed, whole foods will improve with time because you lose your dependence on salt and sugar. Add more beans and nuts to your diet to replace animal products. Try some of my high-nutrient dressing and dip recipes. They use heart-healthy nuts to replace the oils found in traditional dressings and dips.

Level 2 is a reasonable target diet for most people. If you want to lose weight, lower your cholesterol, lower your blood pressure, or just live a long and healthy life, this is the level you should adopt.

LEVEL 3 GUIDELINES

If you suffer from serious medical conditions like diabetes, heart disease, or autoimmune disease, or just want to optimize the nutrient density of your diet to slow aging and maximize longevity, step up to Level 3, where superior nutrition hits its peak. If you suffer from a medical condition that is important to reverse, this is the right prescription for you. If you are on medications and you want to be able to discontinue them as quickly as possible, go for Level 3. It is also the level to choose if you have trouble losing weight, no matter what you do, and want to maximize your results. Level 3 is designed for those who want to reverse serious disease or for healthy people who want to push the envelope of human longevity.

Level 3 is the diet that I use in my medical practice for people who have serious autoimmune diseases (such as rheumatoid arthritis or lupus), or when someone has life-threatening heart disease (atherosclerosis). I prescribe it for diabetics who need to lower their blood sugars into the normal range, or to get rid of severe migraines. It delivers the highest level of nutrient density.

Level 3 includes just two or fewer servings of animal products weekly and concentrates on high-nutrient-density vegetables. Review *Dr. Fuhrman's Nutrient Density Scores* in Chapter 3 to select the most nutrient-dense foods possible. Use green smoothies, fresh vegetable juices, healthful soups, and lots of greens and raw vegetables to make every calorie count.

At this level, you should consume processed foods only rarely. Keep the use of refined fats and oils to a minimum. Nuts and seeds supply essential fats in a much healthier package, with significant health benefits.

YOUR HIGH-NUTRIENT DIET

Knowing how and what to eat is one thing; actually doing it is another. Making great tasting, high-nutrient meals is the best way to overcome any temptation you may have to eat the old, unhealthful, low-nutrient way that was killing you. The easiest way to make mouth-watering recipes is to make the ones in *3 Steps to Incredible Health, Volume 2.* You also can modify recipes you already know, using the guidelines in this book.

Basic high-nutrient guidelines

Here are the things you should concentrate on to assure that you are eating a high-nutrient diet.

1. Eat a large raw salad each day. The amount of leafy lettuce and other leafy greens such as spinach and arugula in the salad should amount to at least five ounces. If you want to jump up to a higher level of excellence, double this quantity of leafy greens.

2. Add other raw vegetables (besides the leafy greens) such as tomatoes, shredded carrots, cabbage, beets, snow peas, or raw broccoli to the salad so the total of raw vegetables for the day amounts to at least twelve ounces of food.

3. Consume a double-portion serving of steamed green vegetables (at least twelve ounces per day). Vegetables such as asparagus, artichokes, kale, collards, broccoli, brussels sprouts, string beans, baby bok choy, and others should be eaten every day. You also can do this by adding these greens to a soup.

4. Eat between one-half and one cup of beans daily in a vegetable soup, on your salad, as an ingredient in a main dish, or in a dip.

5. Eat at least one ounce of raw seeds or nuts daily, preferably in one of the delicious salad dressings or dips you can find in *3 Steps to Incredible Health, Volume 2*. Try to use more seeds and fewer nuts.

6. Eat at least four fresh fruits daily. Try to eat some berries, cherries, or other high-nutrient fruits regularly.

7. Have some freshly squeezed vegetable juice either by itself or as part of your soup base on most days.

8. Measure and control the type and amount of animal products you consume. Do not eat more than one serving of animal products per day, and limit the portion size to less than four ounces (about the size of a deck of cards). As you gain experience, try to reduce the amount of animal products you eat even further. It would be a significant health achievement if you do not have more than one serving of animal products every other day. In other words, whether you have two eggs, chicken in your salad or soup, or a turkey sandwich on whole grain pita, make the next day a strict vegetarian day. Keep your consumption of full-fat dairy very limited, and do not eat processed, barbequed, or salted meats.

9. Reduce and measure your salt intake. Do not cook with salt in the home. Do not eat soup or sauces in restaurants; they are too high in sodium. Always order the dressing on the side, and ask if the food can be prepared without the sauce. If you are using a packaged or third-party prepared food, make sure the sodium content per serv-

ing is the same or lower than the calories. When just starting out, make 400 mg per serving the most you ever eat, and make sure that this is the only sodium-extra food that you consume that day.

10. Get most of your starch intake from carrots, peas, sweet potato, squash, and beans, not from flour products and white potato. Do not eat white flour products. If you're using bread and pasta, use limited amounts, not more than one serving per day and, of course, make sure it is 100 percent whole grain.

11. Limit your consumption of oil to one tablespoon daily. Oil is a fattening, low-nutrient food. If you eat something cooked with oil, make sure you do not use oil on your salad that day.

12. Use *Dr. Fuhrman's Nutrient Density Scores* in Chapter 3 to help you focus your food consumption so you eat larger amounts of raw and cooked vegetables and fresh fruit and smaller amounts of animal products, baked goods, oils, and prepared sweets.

Practice makes perfect

As you now know, the most effective way to properly care for your health is to strive for superior nutrition. To do that, you must stay focused on the nutrient quality of the food you eat. However, I want to reiterate, this program doesn't demand perfection, nor does it mean that you will never eat meat again or that you will never have a slice of birthday cake. It means that your diet has been revamped so that high-nutrient fruits, vegetables, beans, and other foods make up the large majority of your food intake, and that you have the knowledge and skills to come even closer to superior nutrition each day. The instances when you eat meat and cakes will be fewer, but you will undoubtedly find that, with time, those foods are less enjoyable. You may eventually choose not to eat them or other unhealthful foods because you have lost your desire and taste for them and have found healthier options that you enjoy more.

Eating enough healthful food is critical to your success. You will find that when you eat enough high-nutrient food, you no longer desire or even have room for the foods you used to eat. Processed and refined foods offer little in terms of nutrients and phytochemicals. When you eat them, you are losing out on a great many valuable nutrients that your body needs.

What you have read in this book has shown you that there is a whole body of nutritional information that has never been shared with the general public. Even with highly educated health professionals, the power of lifestyle intervention and dietary modifications is hardly addressed because the emphasis is on intervention with pills, drugs, and surgeries. Commercial interests have dominated the nutritional message we have learned to date, and the medical profession has become infatuated with technological advancements. This approach has not only failed to improve the general health of our nation, but it has also resulted in a dramatic explosion of the diseases of nutritional ignorance and pushed health-care spending through the roof without any improvement in healthy life expectancy to show for it.

I hope that you will use the strength of superior nutrition to achieve enhanced vigor and incredible health. Protecting yourself from needless medical tragedy is not only in your best interest, but is a gratifying experience that can bring satisfaction and pleasure to your life. Your success will encourage others to get healthy, too. Perhaps from your example, others will discover how rewarding it is to eat healthfully. The power of the high-nutrient diet is knowledge that we all deserve so that we can make critical choices for our own lives and take back control of our health.

CONGRATULATIONS FOR EMBARKING ON YOUR JOURNEY TOWARD INCREDIBLE HEALTH.

References

1. Fuhrman J, Sarter B, Campbell TC. "Effect of a high-nutrient diet on long-term weight loss: a retrospective chart review." *Altern Ther Health Med* 2008;14(3): publication pending.

2. Svendsen M, Blomhoff R, Holme I, Tonstad S. "The effect of an increased intake of vegetables and fruit on weight loss, blood pressure and antioxidant defense in subjects with sleep related breathing disorders." *Euro J Cl in Nutr* 2007;61:1301-1311.

Ello-Martin JA, Roe LS, Ledikwe JH, et al. "Dietary energy density in the treatment of obesity: a year-long trial comparing 2 weight-loss diets." *Am J Clin Nutr* 2007; 85(6):1465-1477.

Howard BV, Manson JE, Stefanick ML, et al. "Low-fat dietary pattern and weight change over 7 years: the Women's Health Initiative Dietary Modification Trial." *JAMA* 2006; 295(1):39-49.

3. Fuhrman J, Sarter B, Glaser D, Accocella S. "Changing perceptions of hunger on a high nutrient density diet." *Nutrition Journal* 2010;9:51. http://www.nutritionj.com/content/9/1/51

4. Bunyard LB, Dennis KE, Nicklas BJ. "Dietary intake and changes in lipoprotein lipids in obese, postmenopausal women placed on an American Heart Association Step 1 diet." *J Am Diet Assoc* 2002 Jan;102(1):52-57.

5. Sharman MJ, Kraemer WJ, Love DM, et al. "A ketogenic diet favorably affects serum biomarkers for cardiovascular disease in normal-weight men." *J Nutr* 2002 Jul;132(7):1879-1885.

6. Barnard ND, Scialli AR, Bertron P, et al. "Effectiveness of a low-fat vegetarian diet in altering serum lipids in healthy premenopausal women." *Am J Cardiol* 2000 Apr 15;85(8):969-972.

7. Bemelmans WJ, Broer J, de Vries JH, et al. "Impact of Mediterranean diet education versus posted leaflet on dietary habits and serum cholesterol in a high risk population for cardiovascular disease." *Public Health Nutr* 2000 Sep;3(3):273-283.

8. Frolkis JP, Pearce GL, Nambi V, et al. "Statins do not meet expectations for lowering low-density lipoprotein cholesterol levels when used in clinical practice." *Am J Med* 2002 Dec 1;113(8):625-629.

9. Jenkins DJ, Kendall CW, Popovich DG, et al. "Effect of a very-high-fiber vegetable, fruit and nut diet on serum lipids and colonic function." *Metabolism* 2001 Apr;50(4):494-503.

10. Jenkins DJ, Kendall CW, Popovich DG, et al. "Effect of a very-high-fiber vegetable, fruit and nut diet on serum lipids and colonic function." *Metabolism* 2001 Apr;50(4):494-503.

11. Ward S, Lloyd JM, Pandor A, et al. "A systematic review and economic evaluation of statins for the prevention of coronary events." *Health Technol Assess* 2007;11(14):1-178.

12. Tucker KL, Hallfrisch J, Qiao N, et al. "The combination of high fruit and vegetable and low saturated fat intakes is more protective against mortality in aging men than is either alone: the Baltimore Longitudinal Study of Aging." *J Nutr* 2005;135(3):556-561.

13. Hu FB. "Plant-based foods and prevention of cardiovascular disease: an overview." *Am J Clin Nutr* 2003;78(3 Suppl):544S-551S.

14. Esselstyn CB. "Resolving the Coronary Artery Disease Epidemic Through Plant-Based Nutrition." *Prev Cardiol* 2001;4(4):171-177.

15. Schauer PR, Burguera B, Ikramuddin S, et al. "Effect of laparoscopic Roux-en Y gastric bypass on type 2 diabetes mellitus." *Ann Surg* 2003;238(4):467-485; discussion 484-485.

16. Harder H, Dinesen B, Astrup A. "The effect of a rapid weight loss on lipid profile and glycemic control in obese type 2 diabetic patients." *Int J Obes Relat Metab Disord* 2004;28(1):180-182.

17. Barnard ND, Cohen J, Jenkins DJ, et al. "A low-fat vegan diet improves glycemic control and cardiovascular risk factors in a randomized clinical trial in individuals with type 2 diabetes." *Diabetes Care* 2006;29(8):1777-1783.

Ford ES, Mokdad AH. "Fruit and vegetable consumption and diabetes mellitus incidence among U.S. adults." Prev Med 2001;32(1):33-39.

Montonen J, Knekt P, Harkanen T, et al. "Dietary patterns and the incidence of Type 2 Diabetes." Am J Epidem 2004;161(3):219-227.

18. Fuhrman J, Sarter B, Calabro DJ. "Brief case reports of medically supervised, water-only fasting associated with remission of autoimmune disease." Altern Ther Health Med 2002 Jul-Aug;8(4):110-112.

19. Nenonen M, Törrönen R, Häkkinen AS, et al. "Antioxidants in vegan diet and rheumatic disorders." Toxicology 2000;155(1-3):45-53.

Müller H, de Toledo FW, Resch KL, et al. "Fasting followed by vegetarian diet in patients with rheumatoid arthritis: a systematic review." Scand J Rheumatol 2001;30(1):1-10.

McDougall J, Bruce B, Spiller G, et al. "Effects of a very low-fat, vegan diet in subjects with rheumatoid arthritis." J Altern Complement Med 2002;8(1):71-75.

Darlington LG, Ramsey NW, Mansfield JR. "Placebo controlled, blind study of dietary manipulation therapy in rheumatoid arthritis." Lancet 1986;1(8475):236-238.

20. Liu RH. "Potential synergy of phytochemicals in cancer prevention: mechanism of action." J Nutr 2004;134(12 Suppl):3479S-3485S.

Weiss JF, Landauer MR. "Protection against ionizing radiation by antioxidant nutrients and phytochemicals." Toxicology 2003;189(1-2):1-20.

Carratù B, Sanzini E. "Biologically-active phytochemicals in vegetable food." Ann Ist Super Sanita 2005; 41(1):7-16.

21. Hu FB. "Plant-based foods and prevention of cardiovascular disease: an overview." Am J Clin Nutr 2003 Sep;78(3 Suppl):544S-551S.

Campbell TC, Parpia B, Chen J. "Diet, lifestyle, and the etiology of coronary artery disease: the Cornell China study." Am J Cardiol 1998 Nov 26;82(10B):18T-21T.

Fujimoto N, Matsubayashi K, Miyahara T, et al. "The risk factors for ischemic heart disease in Tibetan highlanders." Jpn Heart J 1989 Jan;30(1):27-34.

Tatsukawa M, Sawayama Y, Maeda N, et al. "Carotid atherosclerosis and cardiovascular risk factors: a comparison of residents of a rural area of Okinawa with residents of a typical suburban area of Fukuoka, Japan." Atherosclerosis 2004;172(2):337-343.

22. Hu FB, Willett WC. "Optimal diets for prevention of coronary heart disease." JAMA 2002 Nov 27;288(20):2569-2578.

Esselstyn CB. "Resolving the Coronary Artery Disease Epidemic Through Plant-Based Nutrition." Prev Cardiol 2001 Autumn;4(4):171-177.

23. Gardner CD, Coulston A, Chatterjee L, et al. "The effect of a plant-based diet on plasma lipids in hypercholesterolemic adults: a randomized trial." Ann Intern Med 2005;142(9):725-733.

Tucker KL, Hallfrisch J, Qiao N, et al. "The combination of high fruit and vegetable and low saturated fat intakes is more protective against mortality in aging men than is either alone: the Baltimore Longitudinal Study of Aging." J Nutr 2005;135(3):556-561.

24. Vasan RS, Beiser A, Seshadri S, et al. "Residual lifetime risk for developing hypertension in middle-aged women and men: The Framingham Heart Study." JAMA 2002;287(8):1003-1010.

25. Black HR. "The burden of cardiovascular disease: following the link from hypertension to myocardial infarction and heart failure." Am J Hypertens 2003;16(9 Pt 2):4S-6S.

26. Freis ED. Salt, volume and the prevention of hypertension. Circulation 1976;54:589.

27. Ziegler RG, Hoover RN, Pike MC, et al. "Migration Patterns and Breast Cancer Risk in Asian-American Women." J Natl Cancer Inst 1993;85:1819-1827.

28. Giles LC. "Effect of social networks on 10 year survival in very old Australians: the Australian longitudinal study of aging." J Epidemiol Community Health July 2005;59(7):574-579.

29. Lea EJ, Crawford D, Worsley A. "Consumers' readiness to eat a plant-based diet." Eur J Clin Nutr 2006;60:342-351.

30. Mattson MP, Wan R. "Beneficial effects of intermittent fasting and caloric restriction on the cardiovascular and cerebrovascular systems." J Nutr Biochem 2005;16(3):129-137.

31. Bouchard C. "The causes of obesity: advances in molecular biology but stagnation on the genetic front." Diabetologia 1996;39(12):1532-1533.

32. Weinsier RL, Krumdieck CL. "Dairy foods and bone health: examination of the evidence." Am J Clin Nutr 2000;72:681-689.

33. Sinnett PF, Whyte HM. "Epidemiological studies in total highland population, Tukisenta, New Guinea. Cardiovascular disease and relevant clinical, electrocardiography, radiological and biochemical findings." J Chron Diseases 1973;26:265.

Campbell TC, Parpia B, Chen J. "Diet, lifestyle and the etiology of coronary artery disease: The Cornell China Study." Am J Card 1998;82(10B):18T-21T.

Miller K. "Lipid values in Kalahari Bushman." Arch Intern Med 1968;121:414.

Breslow JL. "Cardiovascular disease myths and facts." Cleve Clin J Med 1998;65(6):286-287.

34. Commenges D, Scotet V, Renaud S, et al. "Intake of flavonoids and risk of dementia." Eur J Epidemiol 2000;16(4):357-363.

Otsuka M, Yamaguchi K, Ueki A. "Similarities and differences between Alzheimer's disease and vascular dementia from the viewpoint of nutrition." Ann NY Acad Sci 2002;977:155-161.

Nash DT, Fillit H. "Cardiovascular disease risk factors and cognitive impairment." Am J Cardiol 2006;97(8):1262-1265.

35. Golay A, Guy-Grand B. "Are diets fattening?" Ann Endocrinol 2002;63(6):2.

36. Maguire EA, Spiers HJ, Good CD, et al. "Navigation expertise and the human hippocampus: a structural brain imaging analysis." Hippocampus 2003;13(2):250-259.

37. He FJ, MacGregor GA. "Blood pressure is the most important cause of death and disability in the world." Eur Heart J Suppl 2007;9:B23-B28.

38. Seals DR, Tanaka H, Clevenger CM, et al. "Blood pressure reductions with exercise and sodium restriction in postmenopausal women with elevated systolic pressure: role of arterial stiffness." J Am Coll Cardiol 2001; 38:506-513.

39. Cook NR, Cutler JA, Obarzanek E, et al. "Long term effects of dietary sodium reduction on cardiovascular disease outcomes: observational follow-up of the trials of hypertension prevention (TOHP)." BMJ 2007; 334(7599):885.

40. Tuomilehto J, Jousilahti P, Rastenyte D, et al. "Urinary sodium excretion and cardiovascular mortality in Finland: a prospective study." Lancet 2001; 357:848-851.

41. Tirschwell DL, Smith NL, Heckbert SR, et al. "Association of cholesterol with stroke risk varies in stroke subtypes and patient subgroups." Neurology 2004;63(10):1868-1875.

42. Roberts JC, Moses C, Wilkins RH. "Autopsy Studies in Atherosclerosis. I. Distribution and Severity of Atherosclerosis in Patients Dying without Morphologic Evidence of Atherosclerotic Catastrophe." Circulation 1959;20:511.

Berenson GS, et al. "Bogalusa Heart Study: A long-term community study of a rural biracial (black/white) population." Am J Med Sci 2001;322(5):267-274.

43. Huxley R, Lewington S, Clarke R. "Cholesterol, coronary heart disease and stroke: a review of published evidence from observational studies and randomized controlled trials." Semin Vasc Med 2002;2(3):315-323.

44. Hu FB, Manson JE, Willett WC. "Types of dietary fat and risk of coronary heart disease: a critical review." J Am Coll Nutr 2001;20(1):5-19.

45. Duwe AK, Fitch M, Ostwald R, et al. "Depressed Natural Killer and Lecithin-Induced Cell-Mediated Cytotoxicity in Cholesterol-Fed Guinea Pigs." J Nat Cancer Inst 1984;72(2):333-338.

46. Composition of Foods—Raw-Processed-Prepared. Agriculture Handbook 8. Series and Supplements. United States Department of Agriculture, Human Nutrition Information Service; Minnesota Nutrition Data System (NDS) software, developed by the Nutrition Coordinating Center, University of Minnesota, Minneapolis, MN; Food Database version 5A, Nutrient Database version 20. USDA Nutrient Database for Standard Reference. Release 14 at www.nal.usda.gov.fnic.

47. Okuyama H, Kobayashi T, Watanabe S. "Dietary fatty acids—the N-6/N-3 balance and chronic elderly diseases. Excess linoleic acid and relative N-3 deficiency syndrome seen in Japan." Prog Lipid Res 1996 Dec;35(4):409-457.

48. Itabe H. "Oxidized Phospholipids as a New Landmark in Atherosclerosis." Prog Lipid Research 1998;37(2/3):181-207.

49. Tucker KL, Hallfrisch J, Qiao N, et al. "The combination of high fruit and vegetable and low saturated fat intakes is more protective against mortality in aging men than is either alone: the Baltimore Longitudinal Study of Aging." J Nutr 2005;135(3):556-561.

50. Fontana L, Weiss EP, Villareal DT, et al. "Long-term effects of calorie or protein restriction on serum IGF-1 and IGFBP-3 concentration in humans." Aging Cell 2008;7(5):681-687.

Fontana L. "The scientific basis of caloric restriction leading to longer life." Curr Opin Gastroenterol 2009;25(2):144-50.

51. Larsson SC, Rafter J, Holmberg L, et al. "Red meat consumption and risk of cancers of the proximal colon, distal colon and rectum: the Swedish Mammography Cohort." Int J Cancer 2005; 113(5):829-834.

Larsson SC, Håkanson N, Permert J, Wolk A. "Meat, fish, poultry and egg consumption in relation to risk of pancreatic cancer: a prospective study." Int J Cancer 2006;118(11):2866-2870.

52. Chao A, Thun JT, Connell CJ, et al. "Meat Consumption and Risk of Colorectal Cancer." JAMA 2005;293:172-182.

53. Sesink AL, Termont DS, Kleibeuker JH, Van derMeer R. "Red meat and colon cancer: dietary haem-induced colonic cytotoxicity and epithelial hyperproliferation are inhibited by calcium." Carcinogenesis 2001;22(10):1653-1659.

Hughes R, Cross AJ, Pollock JR, Bingham S. "Dose-dependent effect of dietary meat on endogenous colonic N-nitrosation." Carcinogenesis 2001;22(1):199-202.

54. Hightower JM, Moore D. "Mercury levels in high-end consumers of fish." Env Health Persp 2003;111(4):604-608.

Mahaffey KR, Clickner RP, Bodurow CC. "Blood organic mercury and dietary mercury intake: National Health and Nutrition Examination Survey, 1999 and 2000." Env Health Persp 2004;112(5):562-570.

55. Mercury Levels in Commercial Fish and Seafood. U.S. Food and Drug Administration, U.S. Department of Health & Human Services. www.fda.gov/food/foodsafety/productspecificinformation. Date accessed: 2/26/10.

56. Ma RW, Chapman K. "A systematic review of the effect of diet in prostate cancer prevention and treatment." J Hum Nutr Diet 2009 Jun;22(3):187-99; quiz 200-2. Epub 2009 Apr1.

57. Cohen JM, Stampfer MJ, Giovannucci E, et al. "Plasma insulin like growth factor-1 and prostate cancer risk: a prospective study." Science 1998(279):563-565.

58. Johnson K. "Dairy products linked to ovarian cancer risk." Family Practice News 2000 Jun 15:8.

59. Melita A, Jain AC, Mehta MC, Billie M. "Caffeine and cardiac arrhythmias, An experimental study in dogs with review of literature." Acta Cardiol 1997;52(3):273-283.

Nurminen MI, Niittymen L, Retterstol I, et al. "Coffee, caffeine, and blood pressure: a critical review." Eur J Clin Nutr 1999;53(11):831-839.

Christensen B, Mosdol A, Retterstol I, et al. "Abstention from filtered coffee reduces the concentration of plasma homocysteine and serum cholesterol—a randomized controlled trial." Am J Clin Nutr 2001;74(3):302-307.

Higdon JV, Frei B. "Coffee and health: a review of recent human research." Crit Rev Food Sci Nutr 2006; 46(2):101-123.

Hallström H, Wolk A, Glynn A, Michaëlsson K. "Coffee, tea and caffeine consumption in relation to osteoporotic fracture risk in a cohort of Swedish women." Osteoporos Int 2006;17(7):1055-1064.

60. Spiegel K, Leproult R, Van Cauter EV. "Impact of sleep debt on metabolic and endocrine function." Lancet 1999;354(9188);1435-1439.

61. Lucero J, Harlow BI, Berbieri RI, et al. "Early follicular phase hormone levels in relation to patterns of alcohol, tobacco and coffee use." Fertile Steril 2001;76(4):723-729.

62. Colantuoni C, Rada P, McCarthy J, et al. "Evidence that intermittent, excessive sugar intake causes endogenous opioid dependence." Obes Res 2002;10(6):478-488.

Rada P, Avena NM, Hoebel BG. "Daily bingeing on sugar repeatedly releases dopamine in the accumbens shell." Neuroscience 2005;134(3):737-744.

63. Link LB, Potter JD. "Raw versus cooked vegetables and cancer risk." Cancer Epidemiol Biomarkers Prev 2004;13(9):1422-1435.

Franceschi S, Parpinel M, La Vecchia C, et al. "Role of different types of vegetables and fruit in the prevention of cancer of the colon, rectum, and breast." Epidemiology 1998;9(3):338-341.

McEligot AJ, Rock CL, Shanks TG, et al. "Comparison of serum carotenoid responses between women consuming vegetable juice and women consuming raw or cooked vegetables." Cancer Epidemiol Biomarkers Prev 1999;8(3):227-231.

64. Key TJA, Thorogood M, Appleby PN, Burr ML. "Dietary habits and mortality in 11,000 vegetarians and health conscious people: results of a 17-year follow up." BMJ 1996;313:775-779.

65. Rolls BJ, Roe LS, Meegns JS. "Salad and satiety: energy density and portion size of a first-course salad affect energy intake at lunch." J Am Diet Assoc 2004;104(10):1570-1576.

66. Unlu NZ, Bohn T, Clinton SK, Schwartz SJ. "Carotenoid absorption from salad and salsa by humans is enhanced by the addition of avocado or avocado oil." J Nutr 2005;135(3):431-436.

67. Steinmetz KA, Potter JD. "Vegetables, fruit, and cancer prevention: a review." J Am Diet Assoc 1996;96(10):1027-1039.

Genkinger JM, Platz EA, Hoffman SC, et al. "Fruit, vegetable, and antioxidant intake and all-cause, cancer, and cardiovascular disease mortality in a community-dwelling population in Washington County, Maryland." Am J Epidemiol 2004;160(12):1223-1233.

68. Bugianesi R, Salucci M, Leonardi C, et al. "Effect of domestic cooking on human bioavailability of naringenin, chlorogenic acid, lycopene and betacarotene in cherry tomatoes." Eur J Nutr 2004;43(6):360-366.

69. Halton TL, Willett WC, Liu S, et al. "Potato and french fry consumption and risk of type 2 diabetes in women." Am J Clin Nutr 2006;83(2):284-290.

70. Jansen MC, Bueno-de-Mesquita HB, Feskens EJ, et al. "Quantity and variety of fruit and vegetable consumption and cancer risk." Nutr Cancer 2004;48(2):142-148.

71. Lau FC, Shukitt-Hale B, Joseph JA. "The beneficial effects of fruit polyphenols on brain aging." Neurobiol Aging 2005;26(Suppl 1):128-132.

72. Gorinstein S, Caspi A, Libman I, et al. "Red grapefruit positively influences serum triglyceride level in patients suffering from coronary atherosclerosis: studies in vitro and in humans." J Agric Food Chem 2006;54(5):1887-1892.

Aviram M, Rosenblat M, Gaitini D, et al. "Pomegranate juice consumption for 3 years by patients with carotid artery stenosis reduces common carotid intima-media thickness, blood pressure and LDL oxidation." Clin Nutr 2004;23(3):423-433.

Duttaroy AK, Jørgensen A. "Effects of kiwi fruit consumption on platelet aggregation and plasma lipids in healthy human volunteers." Platelets 2004;15(5):287-292.

73. Blackberry I, Kouris-Blazos A, Wahlqvist ML, et al. "Legumes: the most important dietary predictor of survival in older people of different ethnicities." Asia Pac J Clin Nutr 2004;13(Suppl):S126.

74. Kris-Etherton PM, Hu FB, Ros E, Sabate J. "The role of tree nuts and peanuts in the prevention of coronary heart disease: multiple potential mechanisms." J Nutr 2008;138(9):1746S-1751S.

75. Hu FB, Stampfer MJ. "Nut consumption and risk of coronary heart disease: a review of epidemiologic evidence." Curr Atheroscler Rep 1999 Nov;1(3):204-209.

76. Ellsworth JL, Kushi LH, Folsom AR, et al. "Frequent nut intake and risk of death from coronary heart disease and all causes in postmenopausal women: the Iowa Women's Health Study." Nutr Metab Cardiovasc Dis 2001;11(6):372-377.

Kris-Etherton PM, Zhao G, Binkoski AE, et al. "The effects of nuts on coronary heart disease risk." Nutr Rev 2001;59(4):103-111.

77. Simopoulos AP. "Essential fatty acids in health and chronic disease." Am J Clin Nutr 1999;70(3):56S-69S.

78. Rajaram S, Sabat AJ. "Nuts, body weight and insulin resistance." Br J Nutr 2006;96 Suppl 2:S79-S86.

Sabat ÃJ. "Nut consumption and body weight." Am J Clin Nutr 2003;78(3 Suppl):647S-650S.

Bes-Rastrollo M, Sabat ÃJ, Gamez-Gracia E, et al. "Nut consumption and weight gain in a Mediterranean cohort: The SUN study." Obesity 2007;15(1):107-116.

Garc-a-Lorda P, Megias Rangil I, Salas-Salvada J. "Nut consumption, body weight and insulin resistance." Eur J Clin Nutr 2003;57 Suppl 1:S8-11.

Meg-as-Rangil I, Garc-a-Lorda P, Torres-Moreno M, et al. "Nutrient content and health effects of nuts." Arch Latinoam Nutr 2004;54(2 Suppl 1):83-86.

79. Lovejoy JC. "The impact of nuts on diabetes and diabetes risk." Curr Diab Rep 2005;5(5):379-384.

Jiang R, Manson JE, Stampfer MJ, Liu S, Willett WC, Hu FB. "Nut and peanut butter consumption and risk of type 2 diabetes in women." JAMA 2002;288(20):2554-2560.

80. Tsai CJ, Leitzmann MF, Hu FB, Willett WC, Giovannucci EL. "Frequent nut consumption and decreased risk of cholecystectomy in women." Am J Clin Nutr 2004;80(1):76-81.

Tsai Cj, Leitzmann Me, Hu FB, et al. "A prospective cohort study of nut consumption and the risk of gallstone disease in men." Am J Epid 2004;160(10):961-968.

81. Liu S, Sesso HD, Manson JE, et al. "Is intake of breakfast cereals related to total and cause-specific mortality in men?" Am J Clin Nutr 2003;77(3):594-599.

Liu S. "Intake of refined carbohydrates and whole grain foods in relation to risk of type 2 diabetes mellitus and coronary heart disease." J Am Coll Nutr 2002;21(4):298-306.

Gross LS, Li L, Ford ES, Liu S. "Increased consumption of refined carbohydrates and the epidemic of type 2 diabetes in the United States: an ecologic assessment." Am J Clin Nutr 2004;79(5):774-779.

Prentice AM. The emerging epidemic of obesity in developing countries. Int J Epidemiol 2006;35(1):93-99.

82. Bravi F, Bosetti C, DalMaso L, et al. "Macronutrients, fatty acids, cholesterol, and risk of benign prostatic hyperplasia." Urology 2006;67(6):1205-1211.

Now that you have learned and put into practice your new high-nutrient way of eating, I hope that you will use it to transform your health. If you haven't read the companion recipe and menu book, *3 Steps to Incredible Health, Volume 2*, I hope you will. It has three levels of menus and all the recipes you need. Once you have prepared a few of my recipes, you can experiment and create your own unique variations.

You deserve a lot of credit for making the effort necessary to step out of the crowd and make a strong commitment to yourself. Each of us has within us a strong inner voice that urges us to survive and to thrive. But most people do not know the best way to respond. You have answered the call, and you know how to respond. Your response will pay big dividends in improved health and enhanced longevity.

Living as we do, surrounded by people who are looking for instant pleasure and effortless solutions to problems, the steady step-by-step diet and health transformation you are undertaking sometimes may seem like an insurmountable task. But as you progress, you will reach the point where renewed joy, vibrancy, and enthusiasm will be your loyal companions. Keep practicing your newly acquired knowledge, and soon it will become your new way of eating and living.

Don't underestimate your body's powerful capacity for self-healing. When high-nutrient eating becomes your *normal* way of eating, you give yourself the opportunity to restore more youthful health and recover from chronic illnesses that many doctors think are "incurable."

Remember, as tremendous as it is, your new knowledge about health is only a first step. You must put this new knowledge into practice and repeat your new beneficial behaviors until they become a part of you. You and I know that it is not easy to develop new habits, and there is no shortcut to developing new skills and expertise. However, if you truly desire to create the "new you," persevere despite any obstacles or temporary setbacks. You don't need to be perfect; you just need to keep on trying. Step-by-step, moment-by-moment, day-by-day, you truly can make your life better and better.

Wishing you much happiness and a long, healthy, and pleasurable life—it can be yours!

NOTES